Helping Relationships in Mental Health

Helping Relationships in Mental Health

Steve Morgan

Community Support Team
Lewisham & Guy's Mental Health NHS Trust
London

Consultant editor
Jo Campling

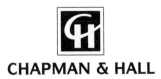

CHAPMAN & HALL

London · Glasgow · Weinheim · New York · Tokyo · Melbourne · Madras

Published by Chapman & Hall, 2–6 Boundary Row, London, SE1 8HN, UK

Chapman & Hall, 2–6 Boundary Row, London SE1 8HN, UK

Blackie Academic & Professional, Wester Cleddens Road, Bishopbriggs, Glasgow G64 2NZ, UK

Chapman & Hall GmbH, Pappelallee 3, 69469 Weinheim, Germany

Chapman & Hall USA, 115 Fifth Avenue, New York NY 10003, USA

Chapman & Hall Japan, ITP-Japan, Kyowa Building, 3F, 2-2-1 Hirakawacho, Chiyoda-ku, Tokyo 102, Japan

Chapman & Hall Australia, 102 Dodds Street, South Melbourne, Victoria 3205, Australia

Chapman & Hall India, R.Seshadri, 32 Second Main Road, CIT East, Madras 600 035, India

Distributed in the USA and Canada by Singular Publishing Group Inc., 4284 41st Street, San Diego, California 92105

First edition 1996

© 1996 Steve Morgan

Typeset in 10/12pt Times by Mews Photosetting, Beckenham, Kent

Printed in Great Britain by Page Bros, Norwich

ISBN 0 412 61750 1   1 56593 437 7 (USA)

A catalogue record for this book is available from the British Library

Library of Congress Catalog Card Number: 95-83014

∞ Printed on acid-free text paper, manufactured in accordance with ANSI/NISO Z39.48-1992 and ANSI/NISO Z39.48-1984 (Permanence of Paper)

To the memory of
Sherman

Contents

Preface

How do you respond to the distress of a man who is sitting before you, in his own flat, towels draped around his shoulders, newspaper wedged beneath the brim of his hat, an upturned frying pan over his hat and a partially filled washing-up bowl balanced on top of the frying pan? He holds the bowl with one hand and a cigarette in the other, while he forcefully proclaims the secret services have placed someone in the flat above to drop radioactive dust down on him all day and all night. To start with, you could offer him a light for his cigarette.

The most likely medical response would be to consider increasing his antipsychotic medicine, though a cursory glance at his medical history suggests that inpatient admissions and large multiple prescriptions of injections and tablets have failed to eradicate the distressing fears that the secret services have occupied the ward above. Perhaps all the increased medication will achieve is to stop him going upstairs intent on retribution. It may even leaden his limbs sufficiently to make his current balancing act too difficult to sustain.

Accepting that the symptoms of distress are very real to him and drugs only achieve minimal alleviation, you endeavour to establish a relationship. Empathic understanding requires that you enquire into the circumstances and the feelings from his perspective. You try not to trivialize or overmedicalize the situation, with the impact of taking power and control away from him. You may even try the diplomatic use of humour to help take some of the potential tension out of the situation: would it not be easier to take your chair into the kitchen rather than bringing your kitchen in to you? What is the record for his kind of balancing act?

Any such humourous repost should be kept short and lead immediately into an attempt to accept and understand what, why and how he experiences his current predicament. Furthermore, you should attempt to

enquire into his wishes, fears, plans, interests and abilities, thus communicating an interest in the person, not the condition.

A focus on the significance of the interpersonal relationship has developed through the intervention of counselling and psychotherapeutic
approaches, with a further impetus created by the change from institutional to community perspectives on care and support. However, the pace
of change in acknowledging the importance of therapeutic relationship
factors in the psychotherapies has not been matched by services offered
to the client group defined as experiencing long-term and severe mental
health problems. They are still primarily treated in the more traditional
sense of the medical model.

The concept of the therapeutic relationship is frequently referred to,
but is often taken for granted as the medium through which the professional process of assessment, treatment and evaluation is performed,
more prominence being given to the diagnosis and specific treatment
interventions. The introduction of case management approaches has
served to highlight the central significance of the working relationship as
a separate intervention in its own right, providing the necessary foundation for the success of other services. Through specific models of case
management, such as the 'strengths' approach, a more client-centred
service can be developed, which challenges the wide-ranging complexity
of needs and offers the potential for real positive change to be achieved
at a very practical level.

Many texts have developed the skills of counselling and psychotherapy, but the skills of engaging in a relationship with people
experiencing severe long-term problems have tended to be overshadowed
in the academic and professional press. The concept of 'helping' relationships is a broad one, extending across supportive, therapeutic and supervisory relationships. This is intended to reflect the broad range of needs
presented by the client group, though it is equally valid to consider an
individual client requiring the focus of support, therapy and supervision
at different times in changing personal circumstances.

Finally, it is important to acknowledge that the type of work envisaged
in this text can be extremely difficult and emotionally demanding for
staff, as well as for service users. The lead established in psychotherapy
services for developing staff supervision is equally relevant to the support, development and growth of staff involved with this client group.

Steve Morgan
May 1995

Acknowledgements

Special thanks are extended to Julie Rogers for typing the manuscript and putting up with any alterations and revisions without complaint; Alan Beadsmoore and Andrew Bleach of the Sainsbury Centre for Mental Health, for their constructive comments and generous access to useful source material, but above all else for teaching me to refer to 'the Sainsbury Centre', not 'Sainsbury's Centre'.

Kate Meads, Chris McCree, Kirt Hunte and Neil Collins of the Community Support Team in North Southwark have given valuable comments on the development of some chapters. Their multidisciplinary backgrounds (occupational therapy, nursing and social work), whilst not necessarily being the main reason for requesting their help, have nonetheless supported my intention that this text should be of value across all professions concerned with the client group. I also wish to acknowledge the contribution of all clients I have worked with in a case management role, for giving me the reasons and motivation to write this text.

Finally, I wish to acknowledge the help and support of the staff of Chapman & Hall, particularly Jo Campling, Lisa Fraley, Sally Champion and Rosemary Morris, for guiding me through the whole publishing process.

Introduction

Human relationships represent one of the most complex processes known. From the beginning of time our biblical, historical, political, natural and cultural development has often been presented through the focus of interpersonal relationships: Adam and Eve, Caesar and Cleopatra, Thatcher and Reagan, Chi Chi and Ann Ann, Morecambe and Wise ... the list is endless. Many of us are fascinated by the trials and tribulations of other people's relationships, hence the popularity of the tabloid press and mass market magazines. We define ourselves, and each other, often by the relationship roles we inhabit: spouse, parent, sibling, offspring, partner, worker/non-worker, gregarious/loner, extrovert/introvert.

Characteristically we tend to define success or failure in terms of the quality of our interpersonal relationships and the quantity of our social contacts. Ask yourself the question whether, today, a classical hermit would be seen as someone with great personal resources and wisdom or as a figure of fun failing in the personal qualities held to be most valuable in human nature?

Similarly, in the development of psychiatry there are frequent references to the nature of relationships as a reflection of the state of mental health. Through the work of Freud, Rogers, Laing and many others we derive theories about relationship factors and mental well-being (Rogers, 1951; Laing, 1959).

Success or failure is frequently measured by the quality of interpersonal relationships and mental health terminology is riddled with phrases that represent poor social adjustment. Many research tools, such as interview schedules and symptom measures, are also heavily weighted to identify problems with interpersonal relationships and the development of social networks (Baker and Hall, 1983; Rosen, *et al.*, 1989).

Much of the literature has focused on aspects of the 'therapeutic relationship' as it is developed from the perspective of the mental health professions (Wills, 1982; Nelson-Jones, 1988; Burnard, 1989; Lloyd and Maas, 1991). It is particularly relevant to psychotherapeutic interventions, where clients are motivated to work on relationship issues that have caused them specific problems that benefit from professionally structured help. However, there has been a more chequered history when we apply psychotherapeutic interventions to people experiencing more severe and chronic forms of illnesses, such as schizophrenia (Gunderson *et al.*, 1984; Wasylenki, 1992).

It is the development of working relationships with the severe and long-term mentally ill client group with which this text is specifically concerned. Chapter 1 will look at a more detailed definition of the clients and their general social context. Bleach (1994) makes reference to:

> ... people who have severe and persistent disturbances of thought, feeling and behaviour as a result of psychotic experiences. They frequently have a wide range of needs across social, medical and personal domains. They often find it difficult to access or accept services that may help them to attain and maintain a maximum level of independence or a reasonable quality of life ... they have usually developed a resentment of service interventions, possibly due to poor experiences, and tend to have little interest in, and often positive resistance to, using the services provided ....

It could be argued that the very organizational structure of mental health services is too fragmented to meet the more complex needs of this client group (Harris and Bergman, 1987). Systems of referral, appointments at set times and places and frequent waiting lists for time-limited scarce resources have done little to encourage the establishment of effective relationships for these people. Deitchman (1980) suggests:

> Economic survival is not successfully dealt with by referral; neither is psychological survival. For the chronic client to survive psychologically, he needs somebody he can have a relationship with, someone he can confide in, someone he can depend on.

For too long, the development of relationships with people who are perceived to be resistant has been largely neglected on the grounds that traditional services view these people either as having low expectations of positive change (Rapp, 1988) or as people who may become too dependent on service providers (Anscombe, 1986). Dependency and personal boundary issues will be addressed elsewhere in the text (Chapter 1).

Rapp (1988) states that it is the relationship that helps to buffer a client against the difficult, stressful and anxious times. It helps them to face the complexities of their interaction with the environment and other people. Kisthardt (1992) reinforces the notion that outcomes experienced by clients are considerably influenced by the quality of the helping relationship, but cautions us to be aware that the building of a relationship takes time and is quite likely to be met initially with suspicion, doubt and uncertainty.

A number of theoretical models and professional processes are examined for their focus on the issues of relationship building (Chapter 2). Case management is seen as a more recent organizational and clinical method developed specifically to target services to the needs of the severely mentally ill client group (Chapter 3). Kanter (1989) suggests that people in this client group are characterized by their difficulty in establishing and sustaining trusting relationships and that this can be addressed by an ongoing personal relationship with a case manager who invests time and effort in understanding the manifestations of their illness, social functioning and social networks. For the strengths model of case management, the relationship aspect of the service is elevated to one of the six stated principles and becomes a central theme of the whole philosophy of the approach (Kisthardt and Rapp, 1989; Kisthardt, 1992). It is my belief that the strengths approach presents one of the most clearly organized demonstrations of how to genuinely focus on the positive aspects of an individual's growth and development, using the intensity of the one-to-one relationship as the prime source of helping intervention. For these reasons, it will be adopted as the basis for much of the presentation of material in this text.

If relationship factors are such a vital element contributing to 'good' mental health, then the processes for establishing and sustaining these relationships, at whatever level, need to be a prominent feature of our professional helping interventions. We may have assumed for too long that clients will automatically respect and trust us for our professional status. The increasing evidence of public scrutiny and litigation, in recent years, suggests that this trust and respect need to be earned rather than expected.

The interpersonal skills of psychotherapeutic interventions have received wide investigation, but the long-term client group may benefit from the informal use of such counselling skills as opposed to the development of the more formal psychotherapies (Chapter 4).

The literature recently directed towards the relationship-building needs of the long-term client group has identified a process of 'engagement' as being a vital first stage requiring its own specific attention (Bleach, 1994). The strengths model of case management is the first of its kind to specify engagement as an individual and separate function (Kisthardt, 1992; Onyett, 1992; Morgan, 1993). The practical development of the engagement process requires an imaginative and creative response to the needs and circumstances of each individual (Chapter 5).

One element of the increased scrutiny and litigation against professional practices has been the growth of an active 'user movement' in mental health. No longer can the professionals simply assess needs on their own terms and provide a service-centred range of provision. Greater dissemination of information, a call for increased choices and a creeping influence of 'market forces' into health and social care have helped to raise the profile of the service users' views. Users are also proposing their own responsive and successful ideas for services, as well as becoming more directly involved in the evaluation of other projects (Morgan, 1993).

Advocacy and user empowerment should not, however, be seen simply as a function of organized groups of service users. It is the responsibility of all service providers to consider how their own relationships with individual users can enhance the empowerment of the client throughout the whole process of interventions (Chapter 6). Once again, the strengths model of case management presents a genuine example of empowering users to direct the process through expressing their personal wants and desires, with the organization of paperwork to reflect this fundamental standpoint (Kisthardt, 1992; Morgan, 1993).

The significance of social context is not simply limited to the experience of severe mental illness and the intrinsic stigmas and disabilities that can accompany the medical conditions. Concerns for race, culture, gender, sexual orientation and mentally disordered offending behaviours have all been seen to compound the psychiatric condition. Whilst each of these facets of the human condition receives deserved debate to reduce the stigma at organizational levels, it is also the shared responsibility of individuals and teams to address these issues through individual relationships, operational policy and professional training (Chapters 7 and 8).

The question of 'supervisory' relationships is twofold: the increasing concerns with aspects of 'risk' have led to further legislation for the introduction of supervision registers (DOH, 1994). Clients at risk of causing violence to others, self-harm or severe self-neglect are subject to placement on registers that will strengthen the powers of treatment and/or recall to hospital. The question of supervisory relationships for clients must also include consideration of the formal detention procedures under mental health legislation and the influences these procedures may have on the helping relationship (Chapters 8 and 9).

With respect to staff, supervisory relationships are a vitally important consideration for addressing personal support and development (Hawkins and Shohet, 1989; Horton, 1993). Working in long-term relationships with very needy clients can be an extremely demanding and stressful task, with high risks of staff burnout. The supervisory relationships can be vital sources of support for addressing specific clinical issues, personal and professional boundary issues, overall workload management and ongoing training requirements (Chapter 9).

A final word of introduction to this text concerns the use of terminology and case material:

Helping relationships — Wide-ranging concept that includes support, therapy and supervision

Supportive relationships — Interventions based on practical tasks and counselling skills in the 'here and now'

Therapeutic relationships — Interventions based on therapy and treatment that are structured, problem orientated and solution focused

Supervisory relationships — 1. Restrictive supervision of clients
2. Supportive supervision of staff

Case material will be used throughout the text to illustrate the content in a way that brings it into a greater perspective of reality. Some case studies will be fully developed to illustrate approaches and some will be short and succinct to highlight specific points of detail.

REFERENCES

Anscombe, R. (1986) Treating the patient who 'can't' versus treating the patient who 'won't'. *American Journal of Orthopsychiatry*, **15**, 26–35.

Baker, R. and Hall, J.N. (1983) *REHAB: Rehabilitation Evaluation*, Vine Publishing, Aberdeen.

Bleach, A. (1994) *'Engagement' Draft Training Module*, Sainsbury Centre for Mental Health, London.

Burnard, P. (1989) *Counselling Skills for Health Professionals*, Chapman & Hall, London.

Deitchman, W.S. (1980) How many case managers does it take to screw in a light bulb? *Hospital and Community Psychiatry*, **31**(11), 788–9.

DOH (1994) *Draft Guidance: Discharge of Mentally Disordered People and their Continuing Care in the Community*, HMSO, London.

Gunderson, J.G., Frank, A.F. and Katz, H.M. (1984) Effects of psychotherapy in schizophrenia: comparative outcomes of two forms of treatment. *Schizophrenia Bulletin*, **10**, 565–84.

Harris, M. and Bergman, H.C. (1987) Case management with the chronically mentally ill: a clinical perspective. *American Journal of Orthopsychiatry*, **57**(2), 296–302.

Hawkins, P. and Shohet, R. (1989) *Supervision in the Helping Professions*, Open University Press, Buckingham.

Horton, I. (1993) Supervision, in *Counselling and Psychology for Health Professionals*, (eds R. Bayne and P. Nicolson) Chapman & Hall, London, pp. 15–33.

Kanter, J. (1989) Clinical case management: definition, principles, components. *Hospital and Community Psychiatry*, **40**(4), 361–8.

Kisthardt, W.E. (1992) A strengths model of case management: the principles and functions of a helping partnership with persons with persistent mental illness, in *A Strengths Perspective for Social Work Practice*, (ed. D. Saleeby), Longman, New York, pp. 59–83.

Kisthardt, W.E. and Rapp, C.A. (1989) *Bridging the Gap Between Principles and Practice: Implementing a Strengths Perspective in Case Management*, University of Kansas, Lawrence.

Laing, R.D. (1959) *The Divided Self*, Tavistock, London.

Lloyd, C. and Maas, F. (1991) The therapeutic relationship. *British Journal of Occupational Therapy*, **54**(3), 111–13.

Morgan, S. (1993) *Community Mental Health: Practical Approaches to Long-term Problems*, Chapman & Hall, London.

Nelson-Jones, R. (1988) *Practical Counselling and Helping Skills,* 2nd edn, Cassell, London.

Onyett, S. (1992) *Case Management in Mental Health*, Chapman & Hall, London.

Rapp, C.A. (1988) *The Strengths Perspective of Case Management with Persons Suffering from Severe Mental Illness*, NIMH and University of Kansas, Lawrence.

Rogers, C.R. (1951) *Client-centred Therapy*, Constable, London.

Rosen, A., Hadzi-Pavlovic, D. and Parker, G. (1989) The life skills profile: a measure assessing function and disability in schizophrenia. *Schizophrenia Bulletin,* **15**(2) 325–37.

Wasylenki, D.A. (1992) Psychotherapy of schizophrenia revisited. *Hospital and Community Psychiatry*, **43**(2), 123–7.

Wills, T.A. (1982) *Basic Processes in Helping Relationships*, Academic Press, New York.

FURTHER READING

Carkhuff, R.R. (1983) *The Art of Helping,* 5th edn, Human Resource Development Press, Amherst, Mass.

Client group and social context

The issue of defining client groups has been at or near the top of the mental health agenda for as long as community care has been the preferred policy for deinstitutionalizing psychiatric services. There are many manifestations of mental health difficulties, but it is not only a task of defining by medical diagnosis (as troublesome as that can often be). Relationships are developed between the nature of the problem and the nature of the prescribed service, but it is not only a task of defining people by the type of intervention. Difficulties occur across very different timescales, but it is not only a task of attributing periods of time as the source of definition.

In his introduction, Onyett (1992) suggests 'Mental health is inescapably a social and political issue reflecting radical social inequalities'. This emphasizes a much broader focus, not just associated with the intrinsic effects of an illness but with its wider social and political implications for disadvantaged individuals. This broader stance is reflected in the emphasis of other writers (Warner, 1985) as well as by the degree of involvement of government in setting the whole policy context of mental health service provision (House of Commons Health Committee, 1994).

This text will be specifically concerned with the people who are often referred to as the 'chronic' client group, as opposed to the implied shorter duration of the 'acute' illnesses. This group of people have presented a particular challenge in terms of formulating an accurate and acceptable definition. The House of Commons Health Committee (1994) have acknowledged that even now ' ... there are difficulties in the way of reaching a definitive description of serious mental illness'. These difficulties are mainly related to the wide range of needs, the constantly changing needs and the transient characteristics of these people.

THE NEED FOR A DEFINITION

Far from just being obsessed with the academic pursuit of clarity of purpose and definition, there are a number of strong reasons why so many people should persist with the task of finding an accurate and acceptable description of the client group. At the simplest level, it is necessary for individual workers, managers and user representatives to communicate a shared understanding of the type of clients they are concerned with. At a more complex level, it becomes necessary for researchers, managers, service planners and government departments to obtain accurate numbers of specific populations in order to record prevalence statistics and to plan service provision within the set budgetary limits.

Furthermore, comparative studies across geographical boundaries require accurate figures based on clear definitions (Schinnar *et al.*, 1991). Access to particular services, e.g. intensive case management, may depend on definitions that closely reflect service access criteria (North Southwark Case Management Team, 1990). Entitlements to specific social security benefits are dependent on meeting set criteria, e.g. middle and higher rates of Disability Living Allowance or the severe disability premium on Income Support. Whilst these latter examples are not synonymous with a written definition of the client group, they provide a basis for the eligibility criteria for such financial benefits to be awarded (Webster *et al.*, 1994; Poynter and Martin, 1994).

In the days before deinstitutionalization the problem of definition hardly seemed to exist. People identified as seriously mentally ill were those admitted to the large and secluded psychiatric hospitals, for long periods of time or even life in many cases. So the only true criterion for definition appeared to be hospitalization (Bachrach, 1988). Deinstitutionalization has produced heterogeneity in the shape of wide-ranging specialist services and a consequent need to match available resources more carefully to identified need. This is why it is necessary to define client groups, to fit into the financial constraints identified above.

LABELS AND STIGMAS

In its crudest form, definition of the client group has grown out of tensions in the form of individual words or short phrases. The tensions have resulted from the different perspectives of the more powerful protagonist groups, vying to impose their separate viewpoints onto the terminology of definition. These groups may be specifically categorized into medical professional, non-medical professional and user organizations.

The result has been a medical preference for phrases such as 'chronic', 'psychotic', 'persistent' and concepts of 'illness'. The user movement strongly challenges the medicalized approach on the grounds that it creates and perpetuates stigma through the labels it attaches to people arbitrarily. It dehumanizes the personal experience of the individual and also denies the more significant periods of time when an individual is 'well' and very capable of determining their own path. The medical terminology has also inadvertently given rise to slang phrases such as 'psycho' or 'schizo', with an inherent burden of social stigma (Chamberlain, 1988).

By contrast, the user movement prefers the use of terms such as 'distress' to more accurately describe the experiences of individuals and also strongly challenges the permanence of diagnostic labels. Many medics argue that the term 'distress' more accurately defines shorter term or acute experiences of other client groups, thus understating the persistent and severe manifestations described by the group of people with long-term mental health problems.

A further compromise, upheld by many non-medical professionals such as psychologists, social workers and occupational therapists, are phrases such as 'continuing care' or 'long-term mental health problems'. They argue a need to acknowledge periods of settled progress rather than persistent illness, but also the vital need to maintain and refocus the goals of support during these settled periods (Pilling, 1991; Morgan, 1993).

There remains no satisfactory single phrase that can adequately define a diverse range of individuals. Whatever phrases I choose to use in this text will quickly find their critics. The user movement is right to remind us all that humanity requires that we acknowledge the individuality of each person and their experiences. Perhaps we should focus less on individual phrases, but be more forthright in pursuing the broader definition of categories solely for organizational purposes and simultaneously focus our active attention on the wants and needs of the individual. In our day-to-day interactions factors of interrelationship should always take precedence over factors of definition.

TOWARDS A BROADER DEFINITION

The complexity of the issue of definition, even at the broad level of categories, is highlighted in the discussion by Bachrach (1988). She suggests that any proposed definition of 'chronic mental illness' should address seven fundamental considerations:

1. the distinction between illness and disability;
2. a clear statement of the psychiatric disorders to be included;
3. the time factor implied by the term 'chronic', including periodicity as well as persistence;

4. allow for future forecasts of disability and illness;
5. minimize the value of hospitalization as a criterion;
6. promote the heterogeneity within the population;
7. acknowledge the range of disability types, e.g. medical, social.

The number of considerations to be addressed clearly points to the inherent failure of words and phrases alone. Bachrach (1988) does, however, concur with the growing credence given to definitions that reflect the interaction of the three concepts of 'diagnosis, disability and duration', though there continues to be a debate on the relative primacy of each.

One example of the interpretation of these elements is provided by Goldman *et al.* (1981), which is also quoted by the House of Commons Health Committee (1994) 13 years later:

1. Diagnosis – schizophrenia, schizoaffective disorder, paranoid psychosis, manic depression or major depression.
2. Duration – at least one year since onset of disorder.
3. Disability – sufficiently severe disability to seriously impair functioning or role performance in at least one of the following areas: occupation; family responsibilities; and accommodation.

'Diagnosis' represents a more traditional medical approach to categorizing patients by detailed description of the symptoms being experienced and relating these to a predetermined schedule of diagnostic categories. Lavender and Holloway (1988) suggest that diagnosis alone, however, will give little indication of the severity of the individual experience.

'Duration' of illness, whilst not the prime element of definition, has given rise to the use of other terminology for categorization (Wing and Morris, 1981; Pilling, 1991), namely:

1. Old long-stay – people typically staying in hospital for five years or more.
2. New long-stay – more than one year but less than five years in hospital.
3. New long-term – not necessarily in need of long-term hospital admissions, but in need of long-term treatment and support that includes hospital admissions.

These three categories have been highlighted in separate studies respectively by Christie-Brown *et al.* (1977), Mann and Cree (1976) and Wing (1982). They give an indication as to the potential subgroupings of client categories, a point which was highlighted by research findings in North Southwark (Sainsbury Centre for Mental Health, 1994).

'Disability', in wider terms of mental, social and occupational functioning, has received growing attention as a prime factor in definitions of the client group (Pepper and Ryglwicz, 1984). The North Southwark Case

Management Team (1990) drew up criteria for inclusion into the service that reflected all three of the above elements, but specifically stressed the value of 'disability' through social functioning and daily living skills impairments:

1. diagnosis of a psychotic illness;
2. depot medication prescribed;
3. more than one inpatient admission in the last 12 months;
4. impairments in either social relations and/or daily living skills;
5. problems in compliance with medication and/or treatment regimes;
6. multiagency user with problems in coordination.

(N.B. Categories 4, 5 and 6 will be given a higher priority.)

Schinnar *et al.* (1991) highlight a further difficulty with the standardizing of definitions for the client group, despite the apparent consensus on including elements of diagnosis, duration and disability. In a study of definitions and prevalence figures for chronic mental illness across several of the states in the US, they found a reasonable degree of consistency in the wording of definitions. A divergence of results was found, however, when studying the different interpretations of the statements for operationalizing definitions to produce prevalence statistics. They conclude with the need to take great care when making any comparisons even when the definitions appear quite similar.

SUBGROUPS IDENTIFIED BY RESEARCH

The Research and Development for Psychiatry (RDP, subsequently the Sainsbury Centre for Mental Health) national case management project included research into pilot studies in four areas of England, including the North Southwark inner city area of London (Ryan *et al.*, 1991; Ford *et al.*, 1993). The initial purpose of the project was to study intensive case management services for the client group experiencing severe and persistent mental health problems (Clifford and Craig, 1988). With this purpose as a core function of the project the research needed to include a detailed description of the client group accepted into the four pilot study areas, in order to determine that they were truly serving the more disabled group they set out to attract.

The Sainsbury Centre for Mental Health (1994) describes the clients who entered into the combined experimental and control groups for the North Southwark study. Sociodemographic and psychiatric history elements of the study are outlined in the left-hand column (CM) in Table 1.1. This set of figures relates to clients identified through the referral criteria for 1990–1. In order to establish the accuracy of this initial case finding process, a replication study was carried out across the North

Southwark area in 1992–3. These results are outlined in the right-hand column (Non-CM) in Table 1.1; they exclude all clients who had already been identified in case management.

Table 1.1 Socio-demographic characteristics and psychiatric history (North Southwark statistics)

	CM n=77 n(%)		NON-CM n=39 n(%)	
Sex				
Male	36	(47)	24	(62)
Female	41	(53)	15	(38)
Diagnosis				
Schizophrenia	63	(82)	36	(92)
Other	14	(18)	03	(08)
Age				
Years (SD)	46	(13.4)	36	(13.3)
Age at first contact				
Years (SD)	27	(9.4)	22	(11.1)
Marital status				
Married	10	(13)	05	(13)
Ever married	25	(32)	08	(20)
Single	42	(55)	26	(67)
Ethnicity				
British Isles	57	(74)	27	(69)
Other	20	(26)	11	(31)
Living arrangement				
Living alone	39	(51)	18	(46)
With relative	27	(34)	15	(39)
Homeless/hostel	10	(13)	06	(15)
Support from carer				
Yes	40	(53)	19	(49)
No	35	(47)	20	(51)
Housing				
No moves (12 mths)	64	(83)	19	(49)
One move (12 mths)	13	(17)	20	(51)
Recent history of violence				
Yes	05	(07)	17	(44)
No	71	(93)	22	(56)

(Published with kind permission of A. Beadsmoore and the Sainsbury Centre for Mental Health)

The most significant outcome of the two studies, particularly in terms of defining the client group, is that two distinct and separate profiles appear, each with equal claims to be representing people with severe and persistent mental health problems.

In general terms, the initial case management project identified a client group older in average age and average age at first contact with psychiatric services. They were also more settled in terms of stable accommodation, with less incidence of forensic histories and/or violence to others. The case management group also tended to be more socially withdrawn and exhibit poorer scores in daily living skills. Conversely, the replication study identified a client group more predominantly male, younger, mobile, volatile, with more of the positive symptoms of medical diagnoses.

The variations are not exclusive to the separate studies, but do point to statistically significant differences between the two study populations. The results serve to highlight the conclusions of Schinnar *et al.* (1991) discussed earlier, particularly the caution over significant differences in interpretation of populations, even when they share the same general definition.

The following two case studies serve to illustrate some of the differences highlighted by the two North Southwark studies. Both people are considered to experience long-term mental health problems, but it is their differences that appear more striking.

Case study 1.1: John (60 years old)

Diagnosis   Chronic schizophrenia; paranoid and depressive elements. Negative symptoms of neglect and withdrawal. Additional chronic physical condition.

Duration   35 year history, with 15 hospital admissions. Generally admitted as a result of severe self-neglect and reduced contact with follow-up services, with incidences of bizarre behaviours. No hospital admissions during last five years.

Disability   Neglectful of hygiene and appearance; lives an isolated, reclusive lifestyle in bed with curtains closed for 23 hours a day. Eats same meal at same café each day. Poor concentration, memory recall and degree of verbal communication with others.

Relationships   Most contact is with café owner and members of statutory services that visit his home. No contact with any family members, neighbours or informal carers. No aspirations to return to day-care services in last ten years.

Case study 1.2: Nathan (32 years old)

Diagnosis   Paranoid schizophrenia. Positive symptoms of a florid nature; auditory hallucinations and paranoid delusional ideas. Frequent use of illicit drugs, viz. cannabis.

Duration   Ten year history, with several hospital admissions. Generally admitted via Mental Health Act sections and/or criminal justice system, following threatening and anti-social behaviours. Four hospital admissions during last two years.

Disability   General life skills and interpersonal relationships become severely disrupted by frequent experiences of persecutory symptoms. Destroys property and displays threatening behaviour towards family, neighbours and service providers. Council tenancy repeatedly under threat due to smashed windows and deliberate flooding also affecting neighbours.

Relationships   Brief periods of positive contact with services and family, displaying a warmth of personality. More frequently suspicious and volatile relationships. Maintains intermittent contact with users of voluntary sector drop-in services. Verbalizes a desire to make a small number of closer relationships with trust and friendship, but not necessarily with service providers.

UNDERSTANDING THE SOCIAL CONTEXT

As we have seen above, definition has an inherent tendency to homogenize the individual into the broader categories of client groups. Efforts to individualize and recognize the circumstances of the single person are aided by broadening our consideration from the 'dimensions of definition' into the additional 'dimensions of social context'. Primarily we aim to concern ourselves with the relationship of the individual person and their own environment. But the notion of 'environment' is a bit too jargonistic and needs to be explained in all its facets of experience (Figure 1.1).

All health and social care interventions take place within a social context. Though intensive case management systems specify the need to acknowledge aspects of individual social context, it is to counselling literature that we have to turn in order to find the rather limited quantity of discussion on the subject (Bimrose, 1993). Figure 1.2 indicates the broader 'societal' dimensions of the environment in which social context is shaped. It is within these discussions that the stigma against mental health is engineered, but also complicated by 'multiple stigma' when we examine the underlying concerns for race, gender or sexual orientiation.

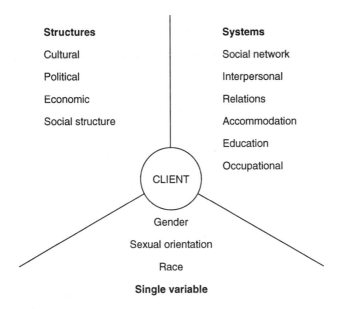

Figure 1.1 Dimensions of social context (based on Bimrose, 1993).

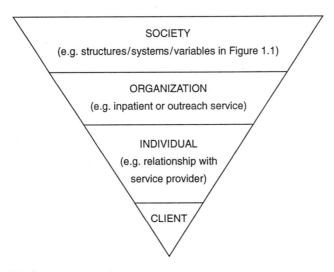

Figure 1.2 Influences on social context.

In addition to the societal dimensions of social context, there are also the influences of the 'organizations' in which we operate, e.g. health trusts and local authority Social Services departments; with their service centred or client-centred outreach philosophies of working. Furthermore, the 'individual dimension' suggests that the separate experiences of the individual service user and service provider, each with their own social context, can influence the nature of interventions and the levels of expectation regarding outcomes of services (Figure 1.2).

Helping relationships in mental health tend to be more commonly framed either within the direct focus of the one-to-one interaction or through the group interaction process. The influence of social context is potentially overlooked or at best relegated to a lowly secondary significance. From such a theoretical standpoint, it is widely assumed that professional interventions need only be learned in the first instance, then applied directly through the working relationship without reference to social contexts. In the field of counselling, this rather simplistic view of the link between theory and practice is increasingly being challenged.

Ivey *et al.* (1987) suggest that the influence of social context is central to the development of theories on which subsequent practice should be based. Frameworks for counselling practice, involving the integration of social context, have been proposed by Egan and Cowan (1979) and Sue and Sue (1990). More radical discussions of the inherent failings of psychotherapy and counselling processes to address the social causes of distress have also been put forward (Woolfe, 1983; Smail, 1987).

Within our development of working relationships with people experiencing long-term mental health problems, it is necessary that a more eclectic viewpoint be adopted in relation to the theoretical frameworks that guide practice. Whether we adopt a predominantly individualist approach to exploring a person's own circumstances and experiences or a more radical standpoint highlighting sociopolitical injustices and stigmas of the system, we still have the central responsibility of establishing a flexible service for individual human beings. It is likely that most of the individuals for whom we are concerned will be seen, in some way or another, as 'victims' of their individual social context, as well as of a broader societal context.

The following case study is presented as an illustration of the wide-ranging factors that may be of some concern in terms of the social context of an individual client.

Case study 1.3: Yanic (74 years old)

Diagnosis   Chronic schizophrenia; paranoid psychosis. Long history of persistent positive symptoms; auditory hallucinations and strongly developed delusional system.

Duration   At least 35 years (no specific information to cover his first 40 years of life). Thirteen-year admission to a special hospital (Broadmoor), with six subsequent admissions to psychiatric hospitals ranging from one to two years duration.

Disability   Self-neglect in most areas of daily living skills, specifically personal appearance and hygiene. Reclusive lifestyle; withdrawn, isolated and suspicious of others, leading to a reluctance to communicate and a preoccupation with symptoms of illness. Deteriorating physical condition due to decreasing exercise and diet, combined with increasing age and smoking.

Social context • Individual: sits alone in living room all day and night (separate room from where his wife lives); smokes cigarettes constantly and interacts with 'voices' which he describes as 'storming' him.
                  • Organizational: community services generally only respond to their own perceptions of crises, e.g. rent arrears and medication. Only attempts to build a relationship were by hospital staff, usually under the authority of legal restrictive powers.
                  • Societal: experiences multiple causes of stigma, due to ethnic origin (Serbian), age and prominent effects of severe mental illness.
                  • Single variable: a Yugoslavian man who came to England after the Second World War, with limited knowledge of English, with his own cultural development, and subsequently isolated by failure of society to naturalize him into the new sociopolitical structures.
                  • Systems: choosing to estrange himself from his increasingly disabled Bosnian wife within the same council flat. No regular contact with his grown-up children. Accommodation of his fixed routine by local shopkeepers and some indirect concern by neighbours fearing he may not be coping well.
                  • Structures: genuinely oblivious to the civil war in his home country, with no knowledge of its effects on his extended family. Living under the conditional restrictions of Mental Health law. Little knowledge of and no sensitive help with housing and benefits entitlements and payments; continues to believe that his council tenancy is in fact 'no-cost' home ownership.

*Development   Referral: only previous community support was a fort-
of a working   nightly 35-mile round trip in a hospital volunteer car to
relationship*   the hospital ward for his depot injection. Conditions of discharge allowed for immediate readmission to hospital if he failed to comply. Other contacts with community

services have been brief discussions about allowing nurses to come into his flat to give the injections and threats to his tenancy because of escalating rent arrears (largely unpaid housing benefit). The result is a psychologically suspicious man becoming even more distrusting of the negative approaches of services.

Method
- Meet informally at hospital ward when he receives depot injections.
- Occasional travelling with hospital volunteer car service.
- Observe the good natural relationship between the client and regular car driver.
- Allow client to make first verbal contact, in his own time.
- Simply respond to client, rather than taking cue for assessment to be progressed.
- Offer help when client explained he was locked out and that his wife was disabled.
- Non-judgemental response to client's concerns over the dirty and dilapidated condition of the flat.
- Accept the client's wishes that home contacts are initially made to help his wife, not him.
- Use basic counselling techniques of listening and attending; offers of practical help only made in relation to client's pace of acceptance.
- 'Understanding' that the psychiatric presentation is a persistent and relatively unchanging factor, regardless of medication compliance; negotiating potential for active support with a parallel concern to ensure client's continued physical safety (failing physical health).
- Negotiate limited joint access with other staff (psychiatrist, general practitioner and community psychiatric nurse).
- Share client's use of words and perception of events, but always mindful to explain alternative viewpoint in an open and non-threatening manner.

Outcomes
- A sensitivity to client's own social context.
- Advocating better help and understanding from statutory services.
- A tentative degree of trust that permitted the case manager to gain access to the flat on all visits, up to a maximum of five visits in a week occasionally.

- Limited access for other staff for assessments and for depot injections at home for ten months.
- Voluntary hospital admission of short duration, on grounds of physical health.
- Hospital ward staff finding client to be more approach-able and communicative than on previous compulsory admissions.
- Physical deterioration causing life-threatening risks in his flat; longer respite hospital admission resulting in reduced quality of relationship with case manager because of the reduced amount of contact.

RELATIONSHIP FACTORS IN SEVERE MENTAL ILLNESS

Beyond the academic approaches to definition of the client group there are the more important subjective experiences of the clients themselves. It is these specific psychological variables that will constitute the 'dis-ability' aspect of the definition and will influence the development of interpersonal relationships. Harris and Bergman (1987) summarize these variables as a lack of stable identity and secure sense of self; scattered and disorganized thinking, becoming easily distracted; easily becoming overwhelmed by external events; sensitivity to stress and an increased incidence of stressful events; and a lack of basic problem-solving skills.

Such a combination of psychological deficits makes the establishing and sustaining of meaningful personal relationships even more difficult, largely as a result of society placing the emphasis on success, ability and conformity to norms of behaviour that are set somewhere beyond the reaches of its psychologically and physically disadvantaged members. Consequently, it should come as no real surprise that the psychiatric literature is steeped in phrases that illustrate the negative relationship qualities attributed to severe mental illness: isolated, withdrawn, lonely, dysfunctional, avoiding, inadequate, defective, rejecting, neglecting, aggressive, repelling ...

It is within the context of such negative emphasis on definition and description, combined with the increasing sophistication demanded by the influences of social context, that health and social care professionals and committed user organizations strive to develop relationships with individuals disadvantaged by the effects of severe mental illness. Whilst acknowledging that medical treatments can rapidly stabilize a physical condition, it is the relationship factors that are widely believed to estab-lish longer term psychological stability, a sense of personal identity and the necessary coping mechanisms for avoiding or dealing with stress.

Much of this text will consider the strategies for establishing and sustaining such relationships, but we must also reflect on the broader relationship considerations of dependency, setting boundaries and risk taking, which together help to define the limits within which the relationship may satisfactorily exist.

Dependency

As in the case of definition of the client group, dependency was hardly an issue while services were organized exclusively in institutional settings. People experiencing severe and persistent mental health problems were expected to live their lives within the confines of the institution and thus be totally dependent on its organizational structures.

With the progress of community care came a growing expectation that people would lead lives of greater independence and thus writers were challenged by the need to explain the nature of change in service delivery that would help to promote this sense of independence (Shepherd, 1984; Pilling, 1991). The notion of dependency subsequently began to assume negative connotations, that maybe the service providers are not doing their jobs properly. Potentially a new iatrogenic condition is being created whereby the services are creating or storing up future problems through the creation of such dependency.

In broad terms, dependency may be seen as a relinquishing of personal responsibility for the fundamental skills of daily living, whether voluntary or involuntary, resulting in varying degrees of reliance on others to make choices and/or perform tasks. The consequence of such a process involves further psychological traumas from the ultimate change or withdrawal of the source of dependency, whether it be an individual or a service. Whilst much has been recorded regarding the notion of physical and/or chemical dependency on alcohol or drugs, very little attention has been drawn to the relational dependency that can be engendered by the method of delivering a service. Furthermore, whilst we may easily acknowledge the potential for dependency in clients, there is also a degree of dependency potential for staff in their clients, as witnessed when people have experienced emotional difficulty in discharging some clients off case-loads.

At the centre, some commentators have proposed the notion of 'normal interdependence' (Rapp and Kisthardt, 1991). This implies that nobody is totally independent in a self-sufficient extreme, but acknowledges that degrees of dependency are both necessary and healthy in our natural interpersonal relationships. The negative connotations of dependency are more recently highlighted as questions against the more intensive models of case management (Chapter 3). Services that focus their approach on the closeness of the user–provider relationship, combined with an all-encompassing comprehensive assessment of needs, will inevitably raise suspicions that the psychiatric institution is merely being perpetuated through the medium of the single service provider.

For this more needy client group, to whom the intensive services are targeted, we may need to acknowledge that some people need a degree of dependency as a result of the disabling nature of their condition. Witheridge (1989) indicates that one of the many training implications for such intensive methods of working is the question of personal attitudes and beliefs towards professional practice and the plight of the client group. We need to accept that degrees of dependency are necessary and normal, but we need to guard against the potential for unhealthy over-dependency. A further intellectual dilemma for many workers is the need to assimilate potentials for dependency with a striving to promote user empowerment (Chapter 6).

One method of managing dependency has been the separation of different professional responsibilities, in line with definitions of core skills, between teams or between members of multidisciplinary teams. Whilst such organization spreads the individual user's contact across a number of service providers, Harris and Bergman (1987) suggest that it creates a fragmentation of service provision which members of the chronic client group fail to respond to and they may thus drop out of contact with needed psychiatric services.

It would appear that in accepting the need for some levels of dependency, we need to build in strategies to our working methods that guard against the potentially dysfunctional levels. One method would be to adopt an approach of 'team responsibility' that requires all team members to perform interchangeable roles with each referred client. This would go beyond the notion of individual relationships for direct contacts but would involve reporting back to some quasi team responsibility through meetings of all team members. Presumably relationships built between, say, one service user and four different team members would reduce the potential difficulties of dependency when one team member leaves the service. The degree of coordination and communication would necessarily have to be very good in order to fulfil this type of function across a whole team service.

Kanter (1989) and Witheridge (1989) refer to the concept of 'titrating' support. The notion relates to a more fluid relationship between the changing level of service user need and the provision of service. However, the prospect of dependency still remains if a single worker is the main focus of that varying service provision. Kisthardt and Rapp (1989) extend this notion into one of 'graduated disengagement' (Chapter 3), whereby the dependency on the relationship with one individual is reduced over a period of time as the changing pattern of needs are accommodated by an increasing network of supports and coping mechanisms.

Boundaries

'Dependency' is a form of 'attractor' and 'boundaries' a form of 'detractor' in the relationship between service users and service providers. It becomes a particular problem if the individual relationship strays from its 'working' function into that of 'friendship'. One of the positive forms of feedback about intensive methods of working has been the client's appreciation that the relationship with an individual worker has gone beyond an expected cold professionalism (Kisthardt, 1992). Whilst the extension of an intensive relationship can provide the benefits of trust, warmth, empathy and even a degree of stability, it is always desired that these developments should be consciously framed within the safety of the care plan. They should not be allowed to slip subconsciously into something that becomes cosy, yet non-productive and potentially destructive to progress for the individual client.

Defence against the potential of such problems takes the form of setting boundaries – the limits which will define the potential of a positive helping relationship. Boundaries are set for several reasons:

1. to identify what constitutes the helping relationship from what shades into friendship;
2. to determine needs for confidentiality, information sharing and expectations of appropriate behaviours;
3. to set realistic expectations on what outcomes may be achieved;
4. to acknowledge that a hierarchy often exists within the relationship, even with positive attempts to promote user empowerment;
5. to determine the need for onward referral and/or discharge from service.

It is important that the nature and scope of such boundaries should be openly discussed between service user and service provider at the earliest possible opportunity. Kanter (1988) indicates the potential for negative transference and countertransference that can result from issues of control and failed expectations when an intensive relationship is established without due regard to the setting of boundaries.

Elements of risk

The assessment of risk frequently receives a high profile as the result of adverse media attention to incidents of a serious nature (Ritchie Report, 1994). Furthermore, attention has been drawn to the issues of assessing potential violence, self-harm and severe self-neglect, through the implementation of supervision registers (NHS Management Executive, 1994). Whilst risk assessment is an essential element of the initial relationship-building process and the development of a good relationship will enhance the subsequent assessment of elements of risk, these specific issues will be addressed in later chapters (8 and 9).

It is of equal importance at this point to consider the more positive aspects of 'risk taking' that may be promoted through the working relationship. For many people within the chronic client group, the taking of risk is not so much a matter of challenging danger as it is a matter of exercising choice and initiating action. For those seen as severely debilitated and possibly highly dependent, the closely developed relationship can be supportive of the idea of taking chances, accepting the failures as being just one part of the learning process. It is about empowering people to act without fear of making wrong decisions, rather than remain inactive because of these very fears. Exercising choice and taking action should be seen as a step-by-step learning process, not as a clearcut issue of success or failure. The relationship can be used to provide a form of safety net and to assess and avoid the danger-laden steps that would involve unnecessary degrees of risk.

Case study 1.4: Mehmet (35 years old)

(Further background details in Chapter 3)

Dependency issues • Parents had separated when Mehmet was only three years of age; he spent large periods of childhood in 'care'.

• Long contact with statutory mental health services had only presented short-term worker relationships, but no settled keyworker to make sense of a fragmented system for him.

• The only long-term consistent relationships had been with two general practitioners at a local medical practice.

• The last few years had seen significant advances aligned with a personal relationship and two consistent workers (case manager and psychiatrist).

Risk issues • One worker leaving the service and the other openly discussing with Mehmet reasons why the second worker may also leave shortly (using an openness to challenge potential dependency).

• Mehmet's responses were to personally increase use of antidepressant, which destabilized his mental state with the effect of rapid mood changes; he also increased his contact with the GPs, up to as much as eight contacts a day on occasions.

- Mehmet rejected the continuing support of his partner and case manager, but openly discussed feelings of rejection with the GPs; also discussed specific symptoms of anxiety with GPs that have consistently intensified at times of stress throughout his personal history.
- Historically, Mehmet's mood swings can raise his suspicions of others, lead to misinterpretation of others and subsequently escalate to indiscriminate acts of violence.

Boundary issues
- Initially determined by actions of Mehmet, within an assessment of risk carried out through a frequent level of contact between formal and informal sources of support; thus the partner and the GPs had daily contact and health service personnel adopted less direct contact.
- The case manager established a stronger coordinating role in support of partner and GPs and informed other health personnel in regular discussions.
- Stability of the episode was followed by a prime focus on learning and teaching Mehmet to understand more about his own reactions to stress caused by actual and potential loss, learning new coping mechanisms and clarifying his expectations of services.
- A need was identified to widen Mehmet's source of contacts for support and thus reduce his apparent reliance on one or two individuals.

SUMMARY

The progressive change from institutional to community care has resulted in a much more fragmented and diverse range of services being provided to clients. The increased flexibility of location and type of service has brought with it a more complex set of eligibility criteria. Resources are necessarily finite, but need to be targeted more clearly to identified user needs. Consequently, there is a growing need for more clarity in the definition of client groups, to match services to user need within the limited resources (Bachrach, 1988).

'Diagnosis, duration and disability' have received growing support as the three main elements of a detailed description of the client group experiencing severe and persistent mental health problems (Goldman *et al.*,

1981). There is less consensus, however, on the relative primacy of the separate elements. Whilst the medical predominance of 'diagnosis' may have held an initial sway, it would appear that the development of widespread multidisciplinary philosophies has promoted the significance of 'disability' in recent years (Bachrach, 1988).

The complexity of definition is intensified when we additionally consider the potential elements that contribute to 'social context'. Whilst definition is more concerned with the broader issue of client group, the notion of social context is a method of further individualizing our description of personal circumstances (Bimrose, 1993).

Addressing the complex needs of an individual requires that we acknowledge the special set of circumstances that define the individual's experience, but some writers also point to the need to adopt a radical approach to social change at the more political and economic level (Smail, 1987).

Within the overall definition of the chronic client group the notions of 'dependency' and 'risk assessment' are identified as important factors in the development of relationships. 'Dependency', like definition, assumed greater importance with the advent of community care. Some people are concerned with the need to facilitate greater independence (Pilling, 1991), whilst others point to the reality of 'normal interdependence' (Rapp and Kisthardt, 1991) and acceptable levels of dependency amongst the more disabled client group (Witheridge, 1989).

Supported risk taking can be a positive outcome of a well-developed helping relationship. It can form the basis of change and growth for the client, but very real concerns about the negative aspects of dependency on a single relationship require us to look closely at strategies for reducing such risk, particularly addressing the appropriate setting of boundaries for defining the relationship.

REFERENCES

Bachrach, L.L. (1988) Defining chronic mental illness: a concept paper. *Hospital and Community Psychiatry*, **39**(4), 383–8.
Bimrose, J. (1993) Counselling and social context, in *Counselling and Psychology for Health Professionals*, (eds R. Bayne and P. Nicolson), Chapman & Hall, London, pp. 149–65.
Chamberlain, J, (1988) *On Our Own*, MIND, London.
Christie-Brown, J.R.W., Ebringer, L. and Freedman, K.S. (1977) A survey of long-stay psychiatric population: implications for community services. *Psychological Medicine*, **7**, 113–26.
Clifford, P. and Craig, T. (1988) *Case Management Systems for the Long-term Mentally Ill*, NUPRD, London.
Egan, G. and Cowan, R.M. (1979) *People and Systems: An Integrative Approach*

to Human Development, Brooks/Cole, California.

Ford, R., Repper, J., Cooke, A. *et al.* (1993) *Implementing Case Management,* Research and Development for Psychiatry, London.

Goldman, H., Gattozzi, A. and Taube, C. (1981) Defining and counting the chronically mentally ill. *Community Psychiatry,* **31**, 21.

Harris, M. and Bergman, H.C. (1987) Case management with the chronically mentally ill: a clinical perspective. *American Journal of Orthopsychiatry,* **57**(2), 296–302.

House of Commons Health Committee (1994) *Session 1993–4 First Report: Better Off in the Community? The Care of People Who are Seriously Mentally Ill* HMSO, London.

Ivey, A.E., Ivey, M.B. and Simek-Downing, L. (1987) Counselling and Psychotherapy: *Integrating Skills, Theory and Practice,* Prentice-Hall, London.

Kanter, J. (1988) Clinical issues in the case management relationship, in *Clinical Case Management: New Directions for Mental Health Services,* (eds M. Harris and L.L. Bachrach), Jossey-Bass, San Francisco.

Kanter, J. (1989) Clinical case management: definition, principles, components. *Hospital and Community Psychiatry,* **40**(4), 361–8.

Kisthardt, W.E. (1992) A strengths model of case management: the principles and functions of a helping partnership with persons with persistent mental illness, in *A Strengths Perspective for Social Work Practice,* (ed. D. Saleeby), Longman, New York, pp. 59–83.

Kisthardt, W.E. and Rapp, C.A. (1989) *Bridging the Gap Between Principles and Practice; Implementing a Strengths Perspective in Case Management,* University of Kansas, Lawrence.

Lavender, A. and Holloway, F. (1988) *Community Care in Practice: Services for the Continuing Care Client,* Wiley, Chichester.

Mann, S.A. and Cree, W. (1976) New long-stay psychiatric patients: a national sample survey of fifteen mental hospitals in England and Wales 1972–3. *Psychological Medicine,* **6**, 603–16.

Morgan, S. (1993) *Community Mental Health: Practical Approaches to Long-term Problems,* Chapman & Hall, London.

NHS Management Executive (1994) *Introduction of Supervision Registers for Mentally Ill People from 1st April 1994.* HSG(94)5. DoH, London.

North Southwark Case Management Team (1990) *Operational Policy: Criteria for Inclusion,* Lewisham and North Southwark Health Authority, London.

Onyett, S. (1992) *Case Management in Mental Health,* Chapman & Hall, London.

Pepper, B. and Ryglwicz, H. (1984) Treating the young adult chronic patient: an update. *New Directions for Mental Health Services,* **21**, 5–15.

Pilling, S. (1991) *Rehabilitation and Community Care,* Routledge, London.

Poynter, R. and Martin, C. (1994) *Rights Guide to Non-Means-Tested Benefits,* 17th edn, Child Poverty Action Group, London.

Rapp, C.A. and Kisthardt, W.E. (1991) RDP Pilot Case Management Project. Workshop on the Strengths Model, Hoddesdon, November.

Ritchie Report (1994) *The Report of the Inquiry into the Care and Treatment of Christopher Clunis,* HMSO, London.

Ryan, P., Ford, R. and Clifford, P. (1991) *Case Management and Community Care,*

Research and Development for Psychiatry, London.

Sainsbury Centre for Mental Health (1994) Conference on 'Providing the Safety Net'. Imperial College, London.

Schinnar, A.P., Rothbard, A.B., Kanter, R. and Adams, K. (1991) Crossing state lines of chronic mental illness. *Hospital and Community Psychiatry*, **41**(7), 756–60.

Shepherd, G. (1984) *Institutional Care and Rehabilitation*, Longman, London.

Smail, D. (1987) *Taking Care: An Alternative to Therapy*, Dent, London.

Sue, D.W. and Sue, D. (1990) *Counselling the Culturally Different: Theory and Practice*, 2nd edn, Wiley, New York.

Warner, R. (1985) *Recovery from Schizophrenia,* Routledge and Kegan Paul, Boston.

Webster, L., Tait, G., Simmons, D. *et al.* (1994) *National Welfare Benefits Handbook*, 24th edn, Child Poverty Action Group, London.

Wing, J.K. (ed.) (1982) *Long-term Community Care: Experience in a London Borough*, Psychological Medicine Monograph Supplement 2.

Wing, J.K. and Morris, B. (eds) (1981) *Handbook of Psychiatric Rehabilitation Practice*, Oxford University Press, Oxford.

Witheridge, T.F. (1989) The assertive community treatment worker: an emerging role and its implications for professional training. *Hospital and Community Psychiatry*, **40**(6), 620–4.

Woolfe, R. (1983) Counselling in a world of crisis: towards a sociology of counselling. *International Journal of Advanced Counselling,* **6**, 167–76.

FURTHER READING

Harding, C.M., Zubin, J. and Strauss, J.S. (1987) Chronicity in schizophrenia: fact, partial fact or artifact. *Hospital and Community Psychiatry*, **38**, 477–86.

Pilgrim, D. (1991) Psychology and social blinkers. *Psychologist*, **2**, 52–5.

2 | Models, theories and processes

Academics and professional practitioners across the whole spectrum of health and social care are concerned with matters of theory. Consciously or subconsciously, wittingly or unwittingly, to varying degrees we are all guided in our day-to-day practice by a variety of theoretical approaches. For some, there is the intrinsic value of investigating and debating the core of theory but even the most practically minded of us will benefit from being aware of our theoretical base. It is only from these solid foundations that we are able to construct practical treatment and support, evaluate different methods of practice, research the efficacy and outcomes of our interventions and communicate the sharing of common practices within a team.

We are in a political climate that is characterized by the influence of financial constraints, economic efficiency and market forces. The laws of accounting pervade all aspects of life, making the demonstration of results even more necessary in order to compete for finite financial resources. Fundamental respect for the virtues of the National Health Service has not been significantly diminished by changing political influences, but like everything else they do now have a price placed upon them.

Notwithstanding the general sense of unease that many people feel about the monetary costing of health and social care, it would appear that attitudes towards medical specialities are once again weighted against sectors such as mental health, particularly the psychosocial approaches. In practical accounting terms it is easier to present costings for the physical, medical and surgical procedures and rehabilitation methods. In psychiatry, it is relatively simple to cost drug prescriptions and hospital bed use but we begin to run into significant difficulties when we attempt to put a financial cost on the development of relationships and the interpersonal psychosocial interventions. How do we begin to cost the long-term intensive support required by a person experiencing the disabilities and disadvantages of chronic schizophrenia? Can we place monetary values on the development of social networks or the support offered to informal carers?

The answers to some of these questions begin to test our moral and ethical, as well as professional, values. Ultimately we must focus more clearly on our underlying theoretical frameworks, either in order to defend the moral value of our services or to present a more fully defined statement of practices for research and evaluation purposes.

THE CONFUSION OF TERMINOLOGY

Whatever the professional background, the language will still converge on the same plethora of terms: models, theories, processes, frames of reference, concepts, theoretical frameworks, ideologies, values, beliefs .... Each can be defined and distinguished as a separate entity, to which end I will refer you to the *Oxford English Dictionary*. For simplicity, I will offer the following distinctions as a basis for the organization of this chapter:

- Model   A simplified representation of reality that explains the relationship of different concepts
- Theory   A system of assumptions and principles used to explain or analyse behaviour patterns
- Process   A series of functions or actions used to organize the method of practice.

Whatever words are used, and frequently interchanged without thought, it is more important to appreciate the link between theory and practice, so that they do not occupy separate and distinct worlds. Furthermore, different theoretical approaches appertain more to individual professionals than they do to the different professions themselves. It becomes futile to pursue an understanding of theories separated by the rigid boundaries of medicine, nursing, occupational therapy, psychology and social work. The existence of multidisciplinary teams often enables a blend of different skills, but frequently team members from different professions are found to share common theoretical frameworks. Conversely, a single profession is likely to present an eclectic range of theories to underpin a broad and flexible range of treatment methods; Finlay (1988) outlines a range of influences on the development of different treatment methods adopted in occupational therapy.

The exception to the above statement would be the medical profession. Psychiatrists tend to adopt a more uniform theoretical framework, widely referred to as 'the medical model'. There are variations on the main theme of this approach, but very few radical practitioners who diverge significantly from it. By contrast, practitioners from the other professions may be exposed to a wider range of theoretical influences, less rigidly scientific in origin and with a lesser sense of upholding the well-established traditions that go with the medical profession. Consequently, the form of training combined with a diversity of beliefs, attitudes, perceptions and cognitions gives rise to a more eclectic approach to practice.

In line with the central focus of this text, I propose to limit the depth of the philosophical inquiry into the different approaches, but to make specific reference to their real or potential influences on the development of client–practitioner relationships. Staff attitudes and perceptions of chronic mental illness, and of individuals within the client group, will greatly influence the extent and nature of the relationship-building function within the overall process of providing mental health services.

THE MEDICAL MODEL

This approach to the treatment of mental health problems is the one with the longest historical traditions and still remains the predominant one today against which all other theories are measured. Its origins in physical medicine are used to support its claims to an objective scientific base, claims which are widely questioned outside the profession (Johnstone, 1989) and less frequently from within (Szasz, 1972). No objectors to the predominant views have been more vehement or justified than the users of services themselves, though the imbalance of power has tended to relegate such opinions to a lowly status (Chamberlain, 1988).

The term 'medical model' primarily refers to a biological view of illness, upholding physical causes as the factors that give rise to the disease process. Johnstone (1989) argues that this viewpoint owes more to the allegiance of the psychiatric profession to the broader medical profession than it does to clear scientific evidence for such causation. Nevertheless, the model proposes the medical identification of symptoms, indicating a formulation of differential diagnoses, which will suggest options for treatment reflecting current medical knowledge. By far the majority of first choice treatments will be physical, i.e. drugs or electroconvulsive therapy (ECT), in line with the scientific aspirations of the profession.

This generalized statement of the model masks a greater diversity of views held within the profession in recent years. One such variation on a theme would be the 'biopsychosocial' medical model. While retaining the central tenet of the biological determinants of mental illness, this all-encompassing approach acknowledges the influences of psychological and social triggers on the underlying biochemistry. Thus, the previously polarized debate of 'genetic vs environment' causes now becomes unified by a less dogmatic view of environmental factors influencing an underlying genetic predisposition to illness. This view conforms more to the 'stress vulnerability' model of mental illness, widely adopted by professionals from a range of training backgrounds. This latter model aims to identify environmental causes of stress, genetic aspects of vulnerability and an understanding of individual coping mechanisms for dealing with such stress (Neuchterlein and Dawson, 1984).

In terms of the relationship building between patient and doctor, the medical model is based entirely on the trust of the 'ill patient' in the professional knowledge and expertise of the medical practitioner. It is not generally seen to be a trust that has to be worked on and nurtured, but more of one that should be immediate and implicit in the role of the qualified professional. This is reflected often in the format of the 'consultation', which may only take a few minutes in the general practitioner's surgery or the consultant psychiatrist's ward round. Longer consultations can be expected in the specialist outpatient appointment at a psychiatric clinic or in the case of a domiciliary visit.

It may be expected that the relationship can grow and develop over many years if the patient is able to see the same GP and/or consultant psychiatrist on a consistent basis. However, the system of medical consultation is still entirely based on the assumption that 'Doctor knows best', so that the patient brings the problem, with the expectation that qualified medical knowledge will provide some form of solution, usually through the physical medium of medication but also with occasional pearls of wisdom in response to some patients' questions.

This view that qualification at the end of training equips an individual professional with restricted knowledge, information and abilities is not held by the medical profession alone. Ultimately, this narrow viewpoint succeeds in maintaining an artificial power imbalance in the relationship between the service user and the service provider. So any potential for change and improvement in the user is limited to the ability of the provider and the potential gains from an empowering of the individual user are effectively denied by the very nature of the relationship.

The position of a power imbalance established through the need for implicit trust in the professional expert does appear to be more extreme and entrenched in relationships with medical practitioners, compared with other health professionals. It may be that the increase in recent years of litigation against all professionals, but particularly doctors, is slowly bringing into question the assumption of implied trust in professional knowledge. Balanced against this slow growth in legal challenges, it must also be acknowledged that the majority of people still feel a sense of safety and security from placing their trust in the skill of the medical practitioner. The consultations, medical treatments and hospitalizations remain valued services for people who frequently find themselves distressed and in need of help.

Within the psychiatric profession there have been a small number of radical dissenters from the traditional theme. Szasz (1972) proposes that disease and illness can only affect the body, so there can be no such thing as 'mental illness'. Involuntary psychiatric treatments are seen as potential crimes against humanity, with no medical, moral or legal justification. He argues that the whole emphasis of treatment should be shifted away from physical sciences to interpersonal communications.

Szasz has been criticized within the profession for holding negatively critical opinions without proposing enough evidence to back his own views. However, the need to focus on the experiences of the individual rather than on the need to describe symptoms and prescribe physical treatments is emphasized by the work of the 1960s 'antipsychiatry movement' (Laing, 1959; Laing and Cooper, 1964; Cooper, 1967). In many respects this work reflects humanistic theories discussed later in this chapter. However, the literature growing from the user movement suggests that antipsychiatry may have been less radical than originally thought, because the emphasis of change in practice lay more in the nature of the consultation and much less in the shift of the inherent power imbalance in the relationship between user and professional (Chamberlain, 1988).

Nowhere is this power imbalance more prominent than in the potential and real use of coercive powers under mental health legislation. Even the built-in safeguards for appeal and review of procedures, the definitions and procedural arrangements are still clearly orientated in favour of the professionals. Recent legislation to introduce 'supervision registers' appears to strengthen the powers more in favour of the doctors. These issues will be discussed further in later chapters.

PSYCHOLOGICAL APPROACHES

Psychology, social psychology and sociology are disciplines that have focused much energy on the development of theories of personality which stress the environmental influences of self and social context (Holland, 1977). Many of the theories have either been reactions to or complementary to the biological emphasis of the medical model.

Whilst the medical practitioners uphold the importance of a rapport in the consultative relationship, in order to elicit a comprehensive picture of the experience of illness, psychological approaches will lay claims to a wider respect for the issues of relationship building. The user–professional relationship is necessary for the full assessment of the individual's circumstances, but also becomes an integral and vital element of subsequent treatment interventions.

I propose to briefly examine the relationship issues that arise from behavioural, psychoanalytic, humanistic and developmental theories.

Basic psychology texts and more specific references to individual theories will give more detailed background information than is possible here.

BEHAVIOURAL THEORIES

Most behavioural approaches are based on the theories of learning pioneered by Pavlov (classical conditioning – respondent learning), and Skinner (instrumental conditioning – operant learning). In essence, they focus on the identification of maladaptive behaviours in the client that need to be changed through the motivational aspects of positive reinforcement or negative punishment. Behavioural theory is a simplified representation of reality that sees human behaviour as a function of learning. A person who is considered unable to function normally has either failed to learn or has adopted socially unacceptable behaviour or behaviour which fails to achieve the appropriate goals (Willson, 1983).

It is the observable behaviour itself that is seen as the problem, not the underlying symptoms of emotional conflict. Adaptive behaviour is expected to help the individual cope more successfully with symptoms and with the demands of independent living. The process is thus:

1. identify the maladaptive behaviours;
2. establish a baseline for treatment;
3. identify the necessary adaptive behaviours;
4. identify appropriate reinforcement;
5. selection of appropriate treatment method, e.g:
   - backward chaining;
   - social skills training (Matson, 1980).

In most respects the relationship between client and therapist in the behavioural approach reflects that previously discussed under the medical model. The power imbalance is similarly upheld through the clear differentiation of a client exhibiting maladaptive behaviours and a trained therapist who will determine the necessary adaptive behaviours, the treatment method and the measurements of successful outcomes. The prescription of physical medical treatment is replaced by the prescription of behavioural changes. The more serious question about the latter point is who is determining the need for behaviour change? If it is the client themselves, then it may be argued that the relationship is one of mutual cooperation. There are occasions, however, when it is the professionals in their capacity as agents of society who are determining the need for change.

In other respects the behavioural approach has been clearly used as a complementary supportive intervention to the primary use of medical treatments. This is particularly evidenced in programmes specifically designed to increase medication compliance, more specifically again in programmes designed to reduce a client's aversion to needles in order to increase compliance with depot injection medications.

The relationship is more frequently based on a collaboration between client and therapist, to achieve jointly agreed goals. It is the mechanics of the method that always reflect the difference in roles, with the therapist adopting a teaching mode and the client required to be receptive to instructions and practise the prescribed new behaviours.

Social learning theory

This particular articulation of behavioural theory emphasizes the importance of environmental or situational determinants of behaviour. Behaviours are shaped through the rewards and punishments perceived through the experience of different interactions in the individual's own environment. The individual learns to discriminate appropriate behaviours in different contexts and maladaptive behaviours can be addressed by social skills training. The main criticism against social learning theory is that an overemphasis on situational influences loses the identity of the individual personality.

Cognitive behavioural therapy

This is a sophisticated concept of understanding behaviours in relation to cognitive processes. By identifying maladaptive cognitions associated with symptomatic thoughts, the potential arises to challenge these thoughts with alternative reality-based cognitions. The use of cognitive behavioural therapy for schizophrenia has steadily grown as an available intervention over the last 15 years (Kingdon and Turkington, 1991). This has reflected the growing assumption that people experiencing psychotic symptoms possess a greater degree of insight than was previously attributed to them. An example of such progress is reflected in work on the modification of delusional beliefs (Chadwick and Lowe, 1990). On the basis of this degree of insight it is thought that people can be helped to better understand what is happening to them and thus to make changes to their own belief systems.

Through its teaching role cognitive behavioural therapy is thought to be able to equip people with effective self-help skills. By developing skills of awareness and recognition through methods of self-monitoring and evaluation, the client is also taught to initiate self-control of emerging maladaptive cognitions through action-based interventions. In relationship terms, the teaching role introduced the inevitable power imbalance between the director role of the therapist and the follower role of the client. The notion of 'therapy' implies more mutual cooperation in the process than would be expected from the more medicalized term of 'treatment'. The empowering influence of cooperation is also reinforced by the progression towards a situation of 'self-help'.

However, care needs to be exercised when considering exactly who is identifying the maladaptive cognitions to be changed – client or therapist. If it is the latter, we return to the thorny question of social control of abnormal experiences.

Personal construct theory

Originally developed by George Kelly (1955), an American psychologist, this is a complex theory of personality which proposes that the individual interprets and predicts events in their world in relation to their own organized system of constructs. The focus is on explaining in terms of the uniqueness of individuals, basing an approach to personality on the ways in which people structure and classify their own social world. These constructs are made up of numerous concepts, e.g. black and white, good and bad, friendly and hostile, which when collectively organized will present a unique picture of the personality of an individual (Claridge, 1977).

The pattern of constructs for an individual will change and modify with experience. Our personality is therefore determined by the way in which we anticipate and respond to events. It is proposed that the thought disorders commonly associated with the experience of schizophrenia reflect a chaotic and loosely organized pattern of constructs, which have a poor predictive value of events resulting in the person responding to situations in a more random and somewhat illogical fashion (Bannister and Fransella, 1980).

In relation to schizophrenia, personal construct theory provides a psychological rather than a biological account. The method developed for the measurement of constructs is the repertory grid technique. This process involves a fairly rigid system of questioning to determine the exact pattern of constructs held by an individual at a given point in time. By examining the ways in which people describe others close to them, e.g. relatives and friends, we have a basis for understanding their individual constructs. The pattern can be plotted on a grid depending on the poles of each construct that the person adheres to. Whilst not constituting a therapeutic relationship in its own right, this specific form of measurement is used with the client to identify maladaptive constructs that subsequent behavioural methods can focus on in the relationship.

DEVELOPMENTAL THEORIES

A number of theories have contributed to what is commonly seen as the developmental approach. Essentially they reflect the ideas that human development follows a chronological process, where each stage is identified by particular attitudes, experiences and acquisition of skills. Disordered behaviour results from abnormal development of the normal milestones or a break in the natural sequence of events. The consequences may take the form of maladaptive behaviours at a particular level or a regression back to earlier stages of development (Willson, 1983; Finlay, 1988).

Mosey (1986) outlines six areas of adaptive skill, each with its own set of subskills. It is believed that the nature of the relationship that develops between two or more people is dependent on the level of subskills attained by each participant in each of the adaptive skill domains. The model of treatment Mosey proposes for addressing levels of skill development is known as 'recapitulation of ontogenesis', which simply refers to a going back over, reaffirming and relearning the skills within one's own process of development.

As with the previously discussed behavioural approaches, the essence of developmental theory involves a teaching and learning relationship between therapist and client. Achievement at one level of subskill by the client results in a progression onto the next level. The significant element of the relationship for the client must once again be their trust in the skill, competence and judgement of the therapist. It is the therapist who largely assesses the level of achievement and plans the appropriate point at which the client proceeds onto subsequent skill levels. It is once again vitally important that a collaborative relationship is fostered to help enhance the client's understanding of the very nature of such progression.

PSYCHOANALYTIC THEORIES

Theories of learning focus on the public personality, primarily concerned with behaviour. In contrast, psychoanalytic theories focus on the private personality, the unconscious motives that direct behaviour (Atkinson *et al.*, 1981). Psychoanalysis was first developed by Freud, who stressed the instinctive and biological aspects of personality. Neo-Freudians, e.g. Klein, have considered personality to be shaped more by people, society and the culture of the individual. Thus we find psychoanalytic theories developing along an axis, with the individual self at one end and the broader social context at the other (Holland, 1977).

Freud's theory of development is based on the notion that humans are driven by the energy that comes from inherited biological instincts, such as hunger, sex and aggression. Psychological tension results from ignoring or repressing these instincts. The four main causes of tension are identified as physiological growth, frustration, conflict and threat. Personality develops through individual responses to these sources of tension.

Freud developed the concepts of id, ego and superego to elaborate his theory of personality development. He discusses the development of defence mechanisms against sources of anxiety and the methods of investigation through 'self-analysis' and 'free associations' (Freud, 1965). However, Freud has been criticized for failing to validate his theory by scientific methods (Holzman, 1970).

The focus of therapy on the resolution of the unconscious causes of emotional pain has tended to make it easier to treat the more insightful and communicative client, predominantly people experiencing neurotic conditions. It has frequently been assumed that people experiencing psychotic symptoms would not benefit from psychoanalytic approaches, due to either a lack of insight into subconscious and early childhood experiences of emotional pain or the potential for these interventions to overstimulate the individual and trigger relapse. Such views have occasionally been challenged through more positive discussions on the application of psychotherapy to schizophrenia (Rogers, 1967; Wasylenki, 1992).

In relationship terms, the psychoanalytic approaches (witnessed through individual or group psychotherapy, transactional analysis or psychodrama) generate a stronger sense of the need to invest in the process of relationship building. A range of counselling skills for engaging the relationship will be discussed in Chapter 4, but the essence of psychoanalysis suggests that the specific relationship is a central element of the treatment outcomes for the client. Trust in the interpersonal attraction is not exclusive to psychoanalytic interventions, but the focus on helping the client to find their own solutions still requires a great investment in the belief of the interpretive and analytical skills of the therapist.

The power of influence is heavily biased to the trained therapist, who must consequently be fully aware of the power and control that potentially could be exerted with such influence, both consciously and unconsciously.

A further aspect of the relationship is the concern with timescales. Different therapeutic interventions will be characterized by different periods of therapy, from the short and focused (cognitive therapy, cognitive analytic therapy) to the much longer, free-flowing approaches. This aspect of time will influence the therapist's approach to the client, in terms of directive or non-directive styles, but will also have a significant influence on the client's perceptions of the therapist, the interpersonal relationship and the nature of the intervention (these influences will be discussed further in Chapters 4 and 5).

HUMANISTIC THEORIES

Humanistic psychology differs from psychoanalytic theories in that it is less concerned with the motivations and predictions of behaviour and more concerned with individual perceptions and interpretations of events. The individual's subjective view of current events takes precedence over the concern with unconscious impulses (Atkinson *et al.*, 1981).

The language of the humanistic movement is that of existentialism and the phenomenological approach. Essentially this relates to the individual's sense of 'being in the world' and is a reflection of behaviour in terms of the perceived present rather than in terms of cause and effect explanations. It is an holistic approach that emphasizes the positive nature of human beings and their pursuit of growth and achievement. However, it has been criticized for the difficulty in validating its central concepts.

Client-centred therapy

The development of this non-directive approach assumes that, given the right circumstances, every individual has the motivation and ability to change. Furthermore, there is an innate tendency for human beings to seek positive change, growth and maturity (Rogers, 1951).

The central elements of the approach are 'self', 'self-concept' and 'self-actualization'. The concept of self is a series of beliefs or a view of oneself which may be partly conscious and partly unconscious. The 'self-concept' held by an individual influences the way in which they experience, perceive and respond to events. The individual will tend to develop in ways which are consistent with their existing structure of self-concepts. The process of expressing and developing the self is one of self-actualization (Rogers, 1967). This idea has been further developed through Abraham Maslow's hierarchy of needs. Self-actualization is seen as the basic motivating force for individuals and a lack of congruence can be identified when a person is seen to behave in a way that is inconsistent with their structure of self-concepts (Willson, 1983).

Willson (1983) suggests that the basic philosophy of client-centred therapy is that:

> Change can be facilitated by a therapist entering into a warm and supportive relationship with the client, in which an 'unconditional positive regard' is shown for the client whatever he says or does. If the client feels respected or valued by another person this allows him to express his less desirable feelings or behaviours, knowing they will be accepted. In doing this he may gain enough support and confidence to examine and accept the more negative aspects of himself or his experience instead of relying on defence mechanisms.

The therapist's role is to act as a sounding board while the individual explores and analyses their problems. The approach differs from psychoanalytic therapy during which the therapist analyses the patient's history to determine the problem and devise a course of remedial action.

This approach has been applied to hospital patients suffering with schizophrenia and the dynamics of the patient-therapist interaction were found to be a significant factor influencing positive outcomes. The therapist is required to demonstrate a clear ability to communicate and to reflect genuine rather than contrived positive regard and empathy.

Solution-focused brief therapy

In line with humanistic psychology, this model of treatment has developed as a way of understanding the unique way in which an individual solves problems and what each person wishes to put in the place of a problem. Problems do not have to be necessarily understood to bring about change. The approach is one of identifying a client's own goals rather than diagnosing or explaining the problem (De Shazer, 1988).

The whole approach focuses on bringing out the client's own strengths and resources, in a way that engenders cooperation rather than conflict in the relationship (Iveson, 1994). In some similarity to the strengths model of case management (outlined in Chapter 3) this approach demonstrates an interest in the client's current and past history of achievement, with a view to establishing their own expression of hopes for the future.

Humanistic approaches view the relationship between client and therapist as a central feature towards facilitating client self-determination. They propose collaborative relationships and uphold the client as the best source of knowledge about their own resources and directions.

The humanistic influence is not just about method; it also impacts on the way we view the whole notion of psychiatric illness, as well as our attitudes towards positive development of relationships.

PROFESSIONAL PROCESSES

The final piece of this 'theoretical jigsaw puzzle' deals with the way in which a profession is able to develop its philosophical base into an organized structure of procedures, to conceptualize its methods of intervention and consequently influence the nature of the relationships between its practitioners and the client group. By way of illustration I will largely refer to my own professional background of occupational therapy.

The whole notion of professionalism is at the heart of how we define our methods of practice; it is also a way of staking claims to unique boundaries and shared territory. It confers a degree of identity and status on the members of each particular profession, but also helps to define the nature and scope of the relationships that may be established with individual service users. A most obvious example would be the legal profession, which immediately conjures up notions of time-limited consultations involving the payment of fees for legal advice and legal representation bound by strict codes of conduct steeped in the traditions of law; or maybe even just a wig and a gavel. We all hold our own stereotyped views of how different professionals may be expected to behave and however inaccurate these views may be, they will already exert an initial power of influence over how we expect to relate with a specific professional.

Occupational therapists lay claims to a variety of psychological influences across behavioural, developmental, psychoanalytic and humanistic theories (Finlay, 1988). Willson (1983) sites five factors that particularly link the profession to a humanistic influence: optimism, opportunity, focus on individual needs, holistic approach and an emphasis on interpersonal relationships. This diversity of influences would suggest a potential similar diversity of approaches to relationship building. However, the ongoing internal debate about the core functions of the profession has only resulted in a widely divergent range of views from outside the profession about what it does and how it does it. Consequently, there is no consistent opinion about the role of occupational therapists from outside the profession, often permitting a perpetuation of unhelpful stereotypes (Stockwell *et al.*, 1987; Joyce, 1993; Harries and Caan, 1994).

Occupational therapy bases its professionalism on its independence from the invasive treatments of nursing or the statutory powers of psychiatrists and social workers. A different aspect of relationship building is thus permissible, with occupational therapists claiming that they have to pay very specific attention to the relationship in order to gain the trust of the individual and subsequent engagement in the activity range that may be offered. Greater attention has to be paid to what the client needs and wants and to their specific strengths and abilities in order to develop a collaborative relationship. Community psychiatric nurses and social workers have been reported as partly sharing this view of occupational therapists taking a uniquely different approach to the client relationship (Brown, 1991).

Whilst there is a clear need to address the development of a good rapport and successful marketing strategies of the product occupational therapy has to offer, there is still the need to address the inherent barrier that professionalism presents in terms of status and power. In terms of organization and efficient use of scarce resources the whole approach is structured into the 'occupational therapy process' (c.f. nursing process in the nursing profession). Figure 2.1 outlines the basic process, but automatically the language, organization, formality and necessary time limits on direct face-to-face contacts will influence the power of the relationship more in favour of the status-bound professional. Willson (1983) suggests that this is not an argument against the existence of professionals, but is a factor that so significantly influences the relationship that each professional should be acutely aware of such influences and be prepared to consider strategies to minimize the potential adverse effects.

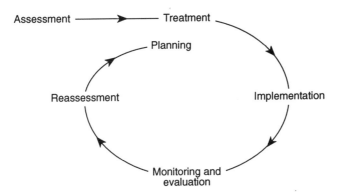

Figure 2.1 The 'occupational therapy process'.

Throughout all functions of the process it is vital to address the quality of rapport between client and therapist. The quality of information forthcoming from the client during assessment will be greatly enhanced by a sense of quality in the relationship. Subsequent successful outcomes are similarly likely to be influenced by the degree of mutual cooperation that pervades the whole process. The question of empowerment will be addressed more fully in Chapter 6, but the sharing of power is dependent upon collaborative information sharing throughout the process.

The potential pitfalls in the process arise from any aspect that will work to reduce the effectiveness of the relationship. If the practitioner undertakes a problem-orientated assessment within an assumption that their training equips them with the sole ability to determine the problems; if the practitioner uses jargon to determine the goals of intervention with scant reference to the client's perception of needs and wants; if the practitioner appears satisfied to narrow down interventions to the limitations of the equipment within a department or office; and if the practitioner evaluates progress from their own observations with little reference to the client's perceptions of change, the consequences of all these strategies are likely to be a poorly formed relationship with a subsequent loss of all the potential benefits of progress that a relationship can support.

The humanistic influences on the occupational therapy profession, combined with a focus on utilizing purposeful activity for promoting personal change and growth, help to guard practitioners against the abovementioned pitfalls. A concern to identify and nurture strengths and abilities in the resolution of problems and conflicts provides a useful baseline for building collaborative relationships.

SUMMARY

The interaction of theory and practice may often be misconstrued. They are not separate and unrelated entities. Whilst the specific function of relationship building may be interpreted as a purely practical task, we need to be aware of the very significant influence that our theoretical base has on our attitudes, behaviours, perceptions and thus on the methods we adopt for developing a working relationship. Approaches may vary from the directive to the facilitative, with very different consequences for the nature and qualities of the ensuing relationship.

The roles of teaching, analysing, interpreting or acting as a sounding board can have different implications for the power imbalance established between the functional therapist and dysfunctional client in the relationship. The whole notion of 'professionalism' in itself perpetuates this imbalance of power through its inherent emphasis on status, definition of expertise, need for organization and management of time and function. Willson (1983) suggests this is not an argument against the existence of professionals, but that there is a need to be aware of the negative potentials on the building of relationships. Furthermore, issues of professional identity should not be allowed to take priority over client needs.

The range of models and theories serves to reflect very different views and points of focus when addressing the needs of the client group. The traditional medical model takes a biological view of illness and disease process, though Szasz (1972) argues against the very existence of an entity such as mental illness. Psychological theories of personality have further developed our focus on public behaviour and/or private emotions.

Motivations for behaviour patterns are variously attributed to learning (behaviourial and developmental theories), unconscious emotional pain (psychoanalytic theories) or perceptions of current events (humanistic theories).

The diverse nature of individual need and presentation within our client group demands that professionals should adopt an eclectic approach to their theory and practice. A particular professional process may reflect a predominant theoretical influence; it may also demonstrate an adaptability to a range of theories, (Willson, 1983; Finlay, 1988), but it remains important for individual professionals working with this client group to be open and adaptable to a range of opportunities and approaches if they are to reflect the broadest sense of individual client need through their working relationships.

REFERENCES

Atkinson, R.L., Atkinson, R.C. and Hilgard, E.R. (1981) *Introduction to Psychology*, 8th edn, Harcourt Brace Jovanovich, New York.

Bannister, D. and Fransella, F. (1980) *Inquiring Man – The Psychology of Personal Constructs*, Penguin, Harmondsworth.

Brown, M.M. (1991) Community mental health occupational therapy: an exploration of distinctive qualities. Unpublished thesis, British Association of Occupational Therapists, London.

Chadwick, P.D.J. and Lowe, C.F. (1990) *Measurement and modification of delusional beliefs. Journal of Consulting and Clinical Psychology*, **58**(2), 225–32.

Chamberlain, J. (1988) *On Our Own*, MIND, London.

Claridge, G. (1977) Personality, in *Introductory Psychology. A Textbook for Health Students*, (ed. J.C. Coleman), Routledge and Kegan Paul, London, pp. 175–219.

Cooper, D.G. (1967) *Psychiatry and Antipsychiatry*, Tavistock, London.

De Shazer, S. (1988) *Clues: Investigating Solutions in Brief Therapy*, Norton, New York.

Finlay, L. (1988) *Occupational Therapy Practice in Psychiatry*, Croom Helm, London.

Freud, S. (1965) *New Introductory Lectures on Psychoanalysis*, Norton, New York.

Harries, P. and Caan, A.W. (1994) What do psychiatric in-patients and ward staff think about occupational therapy? *British Journal of Occupational Therapy*, **57**(6), 219–23.

Holland, R. (1977) *Self and Social Context*, Macmillan, London.

Holzman, P.S. (1970) *Psychoanalysis and Psychotherapy*, McGraw-Hill, New York.

Iveson, C. (1994) Solution focused brief therapy: establishing goals and assessing competence. *British Journal of Occupational Therapy*, **57**(3), 95–8.

Johnstone, L. (1989) *Users and Abusers of Psychiatry. A Critical Look at Traditional Psychiatric Practice*, Routledge, London.

Joyce, L. (1993) Occupational therapy: a cause without a rebel. *British Journal of Occupational Therapy*, **56**(12), 447.

Kelly, G.A. (1955) *The Psychology of Personal Constructs*, Norton, New York.

Kingdon, D.G. and Turkington, D. (1991) The use of cognitive behaviour therapy with a normalizing rationale in schizophrenia. *Journal of Nervous and Mental Disease*, **179**(4), 207–11.

Laing, R.D. (1959) *The Divided Self*, Tavistock, London.

Laing, R.D. and Cooper, D.G. (1964) *Reason and Violence*, Penguin, Harmondsworth.

Matson, J.L. (1980) Behaviour modification procedures for training chronically institutionalised schizophrenics in *Progress in Behaviour Modification*, (eds M. Herson, R.M. Eisler and P.M. Millar), Academic Press, London.

Mosey, A.C. (1986) *Psychological Components of Occupational Therapy,* Raven Press, New York.

Neuchterlein, K.H. and Dawson, M.E. (1984) A heuristic vulnerability stress model of schizophrenic episodes. *Schizophrenia Bulletin*, **10**, 300–12.

Rogers, C.R. (1951) *Client-Centred Therapy*, Constable, London.

Rogers, C.R. (1967) *On Becoming a Person: A Therapist's View of Psychotherapy*, Constable, London.

Stockwell, R., Powell, A., Bhat, A. and Evans, C. (1987) Patient's views of occupational therapy in a therapeutic milieu. *British Journal of Occupational Therapy*, **50**(12), 406–10.

Szasz, T.S. (1972) *The Myth of Mental Illness*, Paladin, St Albans.

Wasylenki, D.A. (1992) Psychotherapy of schizophrenia revisited. *Hospital and Community Psychiatry,* **43**(2), 123–7.

Willson, M. (1983) *Occupational Therapy in Long-Term Psychiatry*, Churchill Livingstone, Edinburgh.

FURTHER READING

Argyle, M. (1983) *The Psychology of Interpersonal Behaviour*, 4th edn, Penguin, Harmondsworth.

Brickman, P., Rabinowitz, V.C. *et al.* (1982) Models of helping and coping. *American Psychologist*, **37**, 368–84.

Davies, R. and Houghton, P. (1991) *Mastering Psychology*, Macmillan, London.

Egan, G. (1990) *The Skilled Helper*, 4th edn, Brooks/Cole, California.

Case management responses

3

It has been suggested that the concept of case management has emerged more as a distinctive and complex model of care rather than as an organizational solution to the problems of adequately coordinating a wide range of existing services (Ryan *et al.*, 1991). Clearly what we are referring to is the complex relationship between an individual client and a worker. Or are we? Maybe it is the relationship between the individual client and a specialized team of service providers? Perhaps it is the relationship between the individual client and the service as a whole? Probably case management is a combination of relationships witnessed through modes of care and of coordination. Or is it?

In the US literature this ideological confusion is widely acknowledged. Bachrach (1989) questions whether the term case management reflects a 'service' or an 'approach'. She suggests that the term is often used without precise definition of its meaning or conversely, that when it has been defined it is used to refer to very different practical operations. Kanter (1989) identifies it as an important function of community support that suffers a lack of consensus about what it actually is or how it should be practised. He elaborates his own definition of 'clinical' case management as a response (Figure 3.1).

Similar confusion has been reflected in, and compounded by, the more recent UK experiences. Ovretveit (1992) states that ' ... The title of case (or care) manager now describes many different roles for organizing care for different client groups. Some case managers are not responsible for all parts of the process of case management; ...' He highlights not just the issue over differences of interpretation, but also the UK debate over the actual title.

Initially, the title 'case management' was adopted in the UK with all its connotations and confusions from its development in the US. It did,

1. ' ... a way of tailoring help to meet individual need through placing the responsibility for assessment and service coordination with one individual worker or team' (Onyett, 1992).

2. ' ... to assist consumers in identifying, securing and sustaining the range of resources, both external and internal, needed to live in a normally interdependent way in the community' (Rapp and Kisthardt, 1991).

3. ' ... a modality of mental health practice that, in coordination with the traditional psychiatric focus on biological and psychological functioning, addresses the overall maintenance of the mentally ill person's physical and social environment with the goals of facilitating his or her physical survival, personal growth, community participation, and recovery from or adaptation to mental illness' (Kanter, 1989).

4. ' ... having a single person responsible for maintaining a long-term supportive relationship with the client, regardless of where the client is and regardless of the number of agencies involved. The case manager is a helper, service broker, and advocate for the client ...' (Intagliata, 1982).

Figure 3.1 Definitions of case management.

however, carry implications of the development of new services for specific needy client groups. The ensuing debate has grown out of a shared user and worker unease with the literal references to 'cases' being 'managed'. Such semantic overtones have sat uneasily with the parallel development of advocacy and user empowerment in service provision, both of which represent some of the most radical and positive advances in recent mental health service developments (Morgan, 1993).

This debate has been reflected in the change of terminology apparent in subsequent policy initiatives. The White Paper *Caring for People* (DOH, 1989) refers clearly to key principles of 'case management'. The NHS and Community Care Act (1990) introduces the concept of 'care management' focusing on the functions of assessment, planning, monitoring and evaluation allied to the purchasing side of services, rather than those of direct provision more commonly associated with case management.

This array of policy language appeared to offer the UK services an opportunity to clarify some of the earlier confusion of definition imported from the US. A clear potential existed for using the term 'care management' in reference to services that focused on coordinating functions, while retaining the term 'case management' for services that focused on the direct clinical and therapeutic functions.

In reality, the semantic debate in the UK has only served, so far, to further cloud the situation through widespread use of the terms 'case management' (Onyett, 1992; Morgan, 1993) and 'care management' (Prance, 1993) often in relation to largely the same clinical entity. For the purposes of this text, I will maintain my own consistency, in some pursuit of clarity, by using the term 'case management' as a somewhat flawed title, but one which relates to the intensive direct approach of relationship building between service users and service providers. Any personal use of the term 'care management' will refer to the 'brokerage' functions currently being adopted by lcoal authority Social Services departments under the guidance of the NHS and Community Care Act (1990). These separate models will be discussed in more detail later in this chapter.

A NEED FOR CASE MANAGEMENT SERVICES

Greater agreement appears to prevail when addressing the question of why such services are needed. The very shift from institutional care to community care required a major change in the delivery of services, particularly when considering the complex multiple needs of the client group often referred to as the long-term mentally ill.

The resulting gloomy picture presented itself similarly in the US and UK, with deinstitutionalization gradually exposing the inadequate responses of the new community services: increasing numbers of homeless severely mentally ill people, high drop-out rates from services and a drift away from using services at a time when individuals appeared most distressed and in need of service support (Rapp and Wintersteen, 1989; Repper and Peacham, 1991). Rapp (1988) suggests that the new community services, based on psychotherapeutic approaches, were not only irrelevant to the biosociological and socioeconomic needs of the more chronic population, but also showed a distinct apathy from many professionals towards the inherent task of providing an effective service for this group.

In summary, Onyett (1992) outlines five general deficiencies that case management services were designed to redress for the client group experiencing severe and long-term mental health problems:

1. a mismatch between user need and service provision;
2. fragmented and discontinuous services;
3. neglect of those most in need;
4. neglect of the needs of informal carers;
5. confusion over service accountability.

WHAT IS CASE MANAGEMENT?

Returning to this vexed question, it would appear that there are as many different statements as there are commentators on the subject. Bachrach (1989) encapsulates the dilemma with the questions: 'How may we define case management for the chronic mentally ill? Is it a service? Is it a clinical approach? Does it consist of brokering, of treatment, or of some combination of these functions?' The simple, though less enlightening answer would be that it appears to encompass all of those. As a result, perhaps it is fruitless to search for the definitive statement, but rather to address its main focus and most clear functions as they impinge on the most important part of the whole puzzle – the service user.

Figure 3.1 details four separate definitions, proposed between1982 and 1992. These definitions are not presented as any attempt to judge and select on merit, though readers may have individual preferences depending on their own experiences or choices for language and simplicity. They are presented in order to draw on common themes and thus shed some light on the purpose of case management. I would propose that the terms 'tailoring', 'assisting', 'facilitating' and 'maintaining', in the context of the respective definitions, refer to the common theme of the relationship between the service users and service providers.

However they may differ in their focus, most discussions on the nature of case management stress the importance of the relationship in order to perform the main functions. The degree of importance or length of time attributed to the relationship differs markedly, but it appears to be the undeniable common factor that underpins the case management process.

In the strengths model the relationship factor is a primary and essential element of the whole process (Rapp, 1988; Kisthardt,1992). Kanter (1988) suggests that ' ... the managerial relationship can be delineated by several characteristics that transcend differences in ideology, professional discipline, and agency setting ...' In the results from an outcome study of a case management project in Toronto, Goering *et al.* (1988) suggest that ' ... the relationship between the case manager and the patient may be the most potent therapeutic factor within the program ...'

Essentially the case management relationship refers to the methods of delivering care through a named individual or team, with the responsibility for ensuring that the full range of clients' health and social care needs are adequately met. Many writers agree on a set of functions implicit in meeting this wide-ranging task, including screening for high need clients, a comprehensive needs-led assessment, individual care planning, detailed implementation of care plans related to stated priorities, advocacy and coordination of services to meet identified needs and a regular monitoring and review procedure.

The relative priorities given to these different functions are the subject of discussion under 'Models of Case Management' later in this chapter and also reflect the different views held regarding realistic case load sizes. Harris and Bergman (1987) suggest that through its stated functions case management is able to become an integrative, rational, proactive and individualized process. They conclude that an essential achievement is its holistic view not only of the individual client, but also of the whole system of treatment and care in which the client is placed. Such a process is able to address the fragmentation of service delivery traditionally witnessed for this client group.

The issue of services being arranged in a somewhat fragmented fashion related to professional specialism and choices presents a particular relationship difficulty for people in the long-term mentally ill client group. Onyett (1992) refers to the inevitable cracks that exist in a service-centred system that plans and organizes itself on the basis of location, age groupings, professions, disability types and even time of day. Morgan (1993) also recounts the failings of a service-orientated organization for this client group and also suggests that establishing and maintaining a wide range of relationships with different service providers is a characteristic difficulty for such people.

In support of the client-orientated focus of case management services, Harris and Bergman (1987) suggest that the coordinated overview of the whole treatment system enables a case manager to bridge potential cracks in the services, thus averting the fragmentation presented by multiple care providers. This focused relationship is able to represent a greater sense of stability to the individual client. Rapp and Wintersteen (1989) reaffirm this point when they propose that the strong relationship fostered between an individual service user and service provider can act as a base of security for a person with multiple and complex needs from the system.

A final comment on the case management relationship, particularly in the intensive clinical-based models, must highlight its potential as a psychological intervention in its own right. Harris and Bergman (1988a), asserting the attributes of a complete case manager, suggest they should ' ... combine the clinical sensitivity and interpersonal skill of the trained psychotherapist with the creativity and action orientation of the environmental architect'. Thus, they uphold the essential need for the interpersonal relationship with the client and the ability to influence change in the wider systems and supports. Ryan *et al.* (1991) develop the significance of the empathy and commitment of the relationship within a broader understanding of stress reactions. They suggest that the case manager combines these skills with those of outreach and advocacy, in order to intervene in situations of stress and high expressed emotion as witnessed through specific early warning signs of relapse.

In summary, the skills of the case manager may be encompassed by the ability to engage a relationship, jointly assess needs with the client and relevant others, in order to develop an individualized package of care that incorporates coordination of other services and supports, in conjunction with the indicated levels of direct work between the case manager and the client. This package of care should then be monitored at regular intervals.

HISTORICAL DEVELOPMENTS

Figures 3.2 and 3.3 outline some of the significant events in the US and UK experiences respectively. Case manager services have developed in other countries, notably Canada and Australia, but I will limit my scope at this point.

Legislation

1964	Mental Health Act – initiating community mental health centres across the country
1974	Supplemental Security Income Program – transferring money from institution to community
1978	National Institute of Mental Health (NIMH) launched the Community Support Program – case management services proposed as a centrepiece

Practical developments

1970	Stein and Test initiate a 20-year longitudinal study at Madison, Wisconsin. Developing a total community living programme
1978–80s	Proliferation of different models of service under the case management title – Strengths model (Kansas) Clinical model (Virginia) Thresholds bridge (Chicago) Community connections (Washington)

Figure 3.2 US experience of case management.

Legislation

1985   Social Services Committee – Services for People with a
        Mental Handicap and People with a Mental Illness

1986   Audit Commission – Making a Reality of Community
        Care

1988   Griffiths Report – Community Care: an Agenda for
        Action

1989   DOH – Caring for People: Community Care in the
        Next Decade and Beyond

1990   NHS and Community Care Act

Practical developments

1980s   Personal Social Services Research Unit (PSSRU)
        study into case management initiatives across client
        groups

1980s   Kent Community Care Scheme – budget-holding ser-
        vices for elderly people

1989   Research and Development for Psychiatry (RDP) –
        pilot projects in intensive case management for long-
        term mentally ill people

1994   Sainsbury Centre for Mental Health Conference –
        introducing title of intensive community support
        teams

Figure 3.3 UK experience of case management.

A most striking contrast appears to be the respective relationships
between legislation and practical developments. In the US, the major
spark for activity followed the National Institute of Mental Health
(NIMH) Community Support Program. A call for case management
projects, without a clear set of guidelines, resulted in many different
models springing up across the states. The work of Stein and Test (1980),
developing a total Community Living Program which dated back to the
early 1970s, has been widely upheld as a blueprint from which other
services have been adapted. However, it is not until the late 1980s that we
begin to see research outcomes and comparative studies of the different

models being made (Harris and Bergman, 1988b; Rapp and Wintersteen, 1989; Bachrach, 1989).

The UK experience is one of much more complex legislation initiating a more specific range of practical developments. Research projects had already been established in line with the early work from the US, studied by the Personal Social Services Research Unit (PSSRU) at the University of Kent in the early 1980s. It was not until the Audit Commission Report (1986) and the Griffiths Report (1988) that the more specific concepts of case management services related to community mental health were referred to. Subsequent legislation introduced the concepts of the care programme (DOH, 1989), an approach to coordinated hospital discharge for all patients, and care management (NHS and Community Care Act, 1990) which establishes local authority Social Services as the lead agency for coordinating community care. The result is a complicated arrangement, already referred to, of budget-holding and non-budget-holding, intensive clinical or coordinating services, with a confusion of titles. The apparent disaffection with the term 'case management' is more recently addressed by the suggestion of intensive community support teams (Sainsbury Centre for Mental Health, 1994).

For further details of the policy contexts and practical developments in the US and UK, including the care programme, see accounts by Ryan *et al.* (1991) and Onyett (1992).

MODELS OF CASE MANAGEMENT

In the comparative simplicity of theory, models of case management can be divided into the 'brokerage' or the 'clinical' categories. The sophistication of practice, however, results in a diverse range of services which lay claim to being models of case management.

Figure 3.4 outlines the theoretical base at each end of a continuum, where brokerage is described as 'administrative' and clinical as 'intensive'. The administrative approach closely resembles what initially became known as care management in the UK. It essentially consists of an assessment of needs, leading to the development of a package of care and a regular monitoring or review of progress. Case managers performing these functions may or may not carry budgets to 'buy in' the required external services to fulfil the package of care (Repper and Peacham, 1991; Ovretveit, 1992).

The intensive model of case management differs in the increased range of functions, contact with the client and amount of 'clinical' input that may be required. Assessment is seen as an ongoing and comprehensive function, as opposed to the more time-limited idea of the administrative approach. Whilst the case manager retains a degree of coordination,

Administrative	Intensive
One stop assessment	Comprehensive assessment
	Outreach
	Intensive direct casework
Coordination of care through keyworker	Advocacy
	Developing natural support
Monitoring and review	Coordination of services through case manager
	Advocacy for services
Case load size: large (35+)	Monitoring and review
	Public education
	Case load size: 10–15

Figure 3.4 Models of Case Management.

monitoring and review related to individual circumstances, they will also be committed to more direct client contact, generally on an outreach basis (as opposed to the more office-based method of brokerage models). The intensive model will also incorporate varying degrees of service advocacy, community networking and education of other agencies and members of the public.

The more sophisticated distinctions between models in practice have been illustrated by Bachrach (1989; 1992). She likens the role of a brokerage case manager to that of an 'enabler', providing the link between client needs and existing service resources. On the other hand, the clinical case manager is seen more in the role of 'therapist', providing much more in the way of treatment through intensive direct contact. The reality becomes more complicated as these two extremes merge closer together (though never entirely) as the enabler is seen to be concerned with treatment issues and the therapist is also concerned with matters of coordination of services.

The clinical and managerial debate is further explored by Harris and Bergman (1987); but for the purposes of this text we are more concerned with the relationship implications for the service user and service provider, which in turn is influenced by the concerns for case load sizes.

Most practitioners of the intensive models agree that it is the investment of time and energy into the relationship with the client that enables people with long-term mental health problems to successfully engage with services (Rapp, 1988; Kanter, 1989). The variety and intensity of functions outlined in the intensive model in Figure 3.4 suggest the need for a long-term relationship. Conversely, the administrative approach presupposes that contact with the client is time limited and task specific.

If we accept the assumption that the client described as being in the severe and long-term category is generally characterized by complex and multiple needs with an underlying difficulty in establishing relationships with others, then the intensive model is the most likely service that will closely respond to their needs, provided that low case loads can be maintained. This approach is also most likely to meet a range of the client's clinical or treatment needs that are often missed by the more fragmented arrangement of traditional services.

Conversely, the statement of functions attributed to the administrative response of a brokerage model suggests that individual client contact is shorter, but leads to the necessary establishment of relationships with providers in a range of other 'brokered' services. This approach essentially provides the overview, coordination and monitoring that may have been missing from the range of existing services. It enables greatly increased case load sizes, but also assumes a degree of cooperation and relationship-building skills on the part of the client. Thus it is suited to many clients, but is a questionable assumption to make if a case management service is designed to target the severe long-term mentally ill client group.

Case load sizes

This issue lies at the heart of the quantity versus quality debate, the question of cost-effectiveness measured against client outcome effectiveness or simply a determination whether the service to be provided is to be service orientated with a wish to meet client needs or genuinely client orientated in its approach. The brokerage models hold some obvious advantages for the service managers accountable to the auditors, in that large or even very large case loads may possibly be accommodated. Rapp (1988) suggests that brokerage models are built on the assumption that a close relationship is not necessary and indicates that some services operate on case loads of 80 or higher. He rightly indicates that a close collaborative relationship cannot be established with 80 people.

One of the main assumptions underpinning the need for case management services is that clients have not managed to engage with impersonal services where large numbers are the accepted norm. As a result, many commentators on intensive models suggest an implicit need for 'low case loads' (Witheridge, 1989; Goering et al., 1988). Onyett (1992) describes in detail a number of projects, the lowest of which works with case loads of only 1–9. Harris and Bergman (1988b) indicate how service planners have expectations of case loads ranging from 20 up to 40, but the evidence from their experience suggests that 12 up to 15 is a realistic limit.

Of course, the numbers game becomes quite hypothetical if we have no system of describing the levels of need of the client group we are working with. However, Harris and Bergman (1988b) also point to other dangerous assumptions, most notably the false premise that client service use decreases substantially after a period of intensive case management. Bachrach (1992) points to the other options of mixing worker case loads to provide a balance of intensities with different clients or using a team approach and selective groupwork interventions. Each of these options needs to be carefully evaluated for its efficacy for the client group. There is always a danger that pressure on services comes before client need, in order to push up case loads or discharge clients. The underlying factor should always be the notion that case management targets the clients with most difficulty and the relationship factor becomes the prime and essential focus for them, not simply for the worker appearing to be resistant to change.

Service models

The sophistication of models already alluded to is borne out by closer scrutiny of actual practice. On the intensive side of the continuum such models as the strengths, clinical and rehabilitation types have been developed in fine detail. The remainder of this chapter will focus on the strengths model as a fully developed exposition of a client-orientated service that places the individual relationship at the centre of practice. Before investigating this model further, a note should be made about the detail of 'brokerage' models. So far, the concept has been applied to the notion of an administrative approach. The work of Brandon and Towe (1989), in the services for people with learning difficulties, outlines a model of independent advocacy that devolves funding and the power of choice right down to the individual service user. In this example, Onyett (1992) suggests the term 'brokerage' is used to define a service that is independent of case management though sharing many similar principles. Once again, we see the confusion of terminology, where different people may use the same term but to describe different functions.

THE STRENGTHS MODEL OF CASE MANAGEMENT

This model of practice has been developed since the early 1980s at the University of Kansas School of Social Welfare. It has become a widely acknowledged model adopted across many states and in November 1991 was introduced through a workshop to the Research and Development for Psychiatry (RDP) pilot case management projects (Morgan, 1993).

A definition of the approach has already been stated in Figure 3.1 (Rapp and Kisthardt, 1991). The UK response to the model has been adequately summed up by Prance (1993) stating ' ... This challenging approach stresses that therapeutic agendas should be set by what the client wants and should reflect the uniqueness of each client's circumstances. Each client has unique personal resources and should work towards his or her own goals ...'.

In relationship terms, the model is a prime example of putting into practice the notion of collaboration between user and worker. The engagement of the relationship is clearly stated as the first vital function of the whole process (Kisthardt and Rapp, 1989; Kisthardt, 1992). Even the use of terminology is specifically targeted to promote the underlying philosophy: strengths, wants, desires, aspirations, individuality, partnership, assisting, valuing, uniqueness. A further distinction of the approach is its emphasis on 'normal interdependence' rather than the frequent focus of rehabilitation on the notion of independence. Whilst some may see this as a further argument in semantics, it serves to illustrate the precise positive detail that this approach accords to the circumstances of the individual. None of us is totally independent, so it makes more sense to stress the reality of interdependence to the clients of our services.

The focus on a client's strengths and abilities is a genuinely radical step away from the more common problem-solving approach, even the problem-orientated approaches that claim to acknowledge strengths as an integral feature of assessment. Weick *et al.* (1989) discuss the narrow view of a client's potential if we maintain our professional focus on the problems we identify. They see the existence of problems as being a limited and unnecessary justification for the presence of professionals, as well as establishing an open acknowledgement of power imbalance between the problem-owning client and the problem-solving professional.

Rapp (1989) suggests that solving problems only returns a person to a position of equilibrium, whereas genuine growth only results from using strengths to exploit opportunities. But he also strongly denies that this is simply a positive reframing of problems; '. . . a strengths perspective is to identify the real and sometimes blatant yet unrecognized talents, histories and aspirations unique to each individual'.

The model itself is based on six principles. I propose to outline each in detail, with illustrations drawn from one specific case study. Figure 3.5 presents some background information about the person who is the subject of this study.

Mehmet – born late 1950s
Turkish Cypriot origin. Parents separated when he was three years old. Moved from Cyprus to UK at age of ten to live with his father and stepmother.

Psychiatric history
- Fourteen hospital admissions between 1977 and 1992
- Frequent admissions to locked wards via criminal justice system
- Diagnosis of schizophrenia, with history of abusing cannabis and alcohol
- Treated for varying periods of time on neuroleptic medications and carbamazepine and lithium

Forensic history
- Ten charges of assault causing actual bodily harm between 1983 and 1991
- Two prison sentences served, with additional periods remanded in prison and on Sections of the 1983 Mental Health Act

Housing history
- Lived with father and stepmother up to 1983
- Between 1983 and 1990 he had separate local authority tenancies, interrupted by frequent hospital and prison stays
- 1991 made officially homeless by Housing Department on grounds of arson

---

Figure 3.5 Background case study material.

Principle 1: The focus of the helping process is upon the client's strengths, interests, abilities and competencies, not upon their deficits, weaknesses or problems.

The basis of this principle is that, given choice, we all prefer to spend time doing the things we are good at and those that we enjoy. We avoid the things we are not good at or at least where we perceive the potential for failure. Yet frequently in our work with clients we attempt to get them to look at their problems, their weaknesses and failings.

If we approach each client with a view to assessing their problems, particularly somebody categorized as suffering severe and long-term mental health problems, the list makes for a rather depressing picture of failure. If the client is not depressed at the start of the process they have every right to be at the end. Furthermore, our terminology tends to present problems as generalized statements: poor motivation, poor personal hygiene, mild learning difficulties, self-neglect, social isolation. These statements tend to further categorize people into stereotyped groups; there is no sense of the uniqueness of an individual.

If, on the other hand, we focus our attention on the person's strengths, achievements, actual and potential resources and their desires for the future, we begin to build a picture of a unique set of circumstances specific to one individual. A genuinely positive focus on a person's past, present and future also promotes more favourable conditions for motivation to achieve some of the personal goals the client is encouraged to express.

Mehmet

Despite an obvious history of difficulties that had been recurring with regularity, Mehmet was encouraged by the case management process to focus on:

- aspects of his personality that could generate warmth towards others, which had helped him previously and currently to establish relationships with some people;
- a desire to improve health and fitness through physical exercise, including weight-training;
- a desire to prove that he could cope with the responsibility of a new flat, with help from others.

Principle 2: All clients have the capacity to learn, grow and change.

This principle is based on the assumption that individual clients do not lose their hopes and their dreams as a consequence of the diagnosis of a severe mental illness but is also as much about the attitudes of the staff as it is about the attitudes of clients.

Rapp (1988) suggests that the mental health system has managed to 'institutionalize low expectations' of people in this client group. Through our training and experience we come to see the burden of problems as a block to any change and growth. Staff who hold such low expectations of clients will communicate as much to them and hence find it impossible to facilitate and support a client's achievement of their own goals and dreams.

In reality, clients should be encouraged to set realistically achievable goals as steps towards their greater wishes. They should be encouraged to take risks as positive attempts to succeed and to accept some failure as a natural part of the learning process.

Mehmet

Wishes to improve his standard of spoken and written English, to be more clearly understood by others. He sees part of his own frustrations and anger as being a response to his misunderstanding of others and also a perception of other people being impatient with his slow rate of learning. Mehmet shows a frequent desire to learn more about his own psychiatric condition, to make some sense of the strange thoughts and behaviours that severely affected his life. He frequently wishes to verbalize his own history as he sees it.

Principle 3: The client is viewed as the director of the case management helping process.

This principle forms an important aspect of empowering service users to take more control of their own lives and to be actively determining the form and direction that their experiences of case management should take. By following this principle we uphold the ideas of 'working with' the client, rather than a 'doing for' paternalistic stance. We are helping to promote a sense of self-determination.

When encouraging the clients to say what they want, we must take the information we receive seriously and not ignore any differences from our own service-centred agendas. Once again there is an element of positive risk taking, a sense of going with the flow, but in a manner that realistic goals can be set and subsequently built upon through a genuine sense of collaboration.

Mehmet

When he was initially detained on a locked ward with intensive medical supervision, the case manager was the one professional that Mehmet was able to instruct to work immediately on his own priorities, rather than having the service priorities of medical and nursing care reiterated back to him. In the circumstances, Mehmet saw his lack of housing and his enforced homeless status as the main priority for the case manager to work on. Subsequently, since his discharge to a new council tenancy, Mehmet uses formal and informal reviews with the case manager to express any changing priorities.

Principle 4: The client–case manager relationship becomes a primary and essential partnership

Unlike the administrative models of case management, the strengths model clearly states that the central element of the work is based on a stable, long-term relationship between an individual client and a case manager. The quality of that relationship is seen as crucial to working effectively, both in terms of aiming for the positive achievements and for acting as a buffer when things are not going so well.

Deitchman (1980) suggests that what the long-term client needs is a 'travel companion' not a 'travel agent' – somebody who will be with them to share experiences, not just someone who will give the directions and then leave them to it. This necessitates active work on behalf of the case manager to engage the relationship through self-disclosure and offering a service that meets the requirements of the client.

Mehmet

For much of the first 18 months the relationship was of a poor quality. Mehmet was largely detained in hospital or remanded in prison, angry with the continuation of the negative circumstances and distrustful of anyone suggesting they had a different service to offer. He had set the case manager the difficult sole task of resolving his housing predicament. Successful resolution of the challenge, combined with other demonstrations of advocacy for financial benefits and outreach work with other available supports, all resulted in the development of a working partnership. Mehmet now feels able to reciprocate genuine warmth, hospitality and occasional concern for the case manager.

Principle 5: The case management helping process takes on an outreach perspective.

This principle is again linked to the notion of further empowering the user, by giving them the choice as to where the work should take place. Most people in this client group express concerns about the need for them to attend service facilities largely by appointment. Non-attendance is a problem. Thus, the principle of outreach is a method of shifting the focus of responsibility from a service-centred plan of organization to something more client centred.

A further advantage of operating an outreach service is the greater amount of knowledge that can be gathered about the client and their local community. Support and care plans can be made more realistic if they relate directly to the world inhabited by the client, rather than the artificial setting of most service bases.

A note of caution and flexibility needs to be introduced with this principle. In the interests of personal safety, workers should be aware of any vital information about the client, carers or the local environment before they agree to a situation that puts them in unnecessary risk. Conversely, some clients will feel safer and more comfortable with the initial meetings taking place at a clinic or mental health centre.

Mehmet

For much of the first 12 months meetings occurred at hospital wards, locked units and the Accident and Emergency department of a local hospital. The changing focus of the work required meetings at housing department offices, solicitors' offices and cafés. More recently meetings occur at an education centre and generally at the client's own home.

Additional outreach work at an early stage involved contact and support for relatives and his partner.

Principle 6: The entire community is viewed as an oasis of potential resources rather than as an obstacle. Natural community resources should be considered before segregated mental health services.

A frequent concern expressed by beleaguered mental health professionals is the lack of community mental health services available for their clients to be referred to. The basis of this principle in the strengths model is that people are not integrated into their local community if all you have done is place them full-time in the hands of segregated mental health services. In this situation, the client has only truly been integrated into their 'psychiatric community' and all the same problems of stigmatization are likely to abound.

The principle of using the natural community resources is based on a belief that there are many helpful and understanding people willing to offer support to needy individuals. They are not generally as vocal as those who perpetuate stigmatization and finding them requires a degree of imaginative thinking, knowing the community and above all else, proactive outreach work alongside the client. As with all aspects of this work, it is time consuming, risk taking and will not always be successful, but it extends the bounds of knowledge way beyond what can be achieved only at an office base.

Mehmet

During 17 years of contact with psychiatric services Mehmet has steadfastly refused to accept contact with community mental health day-care services during the periods he has been discharged into the community. Family and friends within the Turkish Cypriot community cafés have always been a higher priority.

More recently he has joined a community literacy scheme to improve his English and regularly attends a local gymnasium. Mental health resources could have been found to meet those needs, but that was never on Mehmet's agenda and would certainly have provided a poorer standard of service for him.

Mehmet has recently been on holiday – not for him a week with a group of people from a mental health centre visiting a UK tourist spot; he has been with his partner for two weeks to Turkey, even remembering to bring back some real Turkish Delight confectionery for his case manager and consultant psychiatrist.

FUNCTIONS OF THE STRENGTHS MODEL

Figure 3.6 outlines the main functions of the strengths model of case management. The purpose of these functions is to show how the six principles become observable activities (Kisthardt and Rapp, 1989). In common with many articulations of a professional process, e.g. nursing or occupational therapy processes, it is not to be seen as a strictly linear entity, but as a fluid pattern that evolves, changes and feeds back information into its early parts.

- Engagement
- Assessment (wants-based)
- Care planning (needs-based)
- Implementation (including 'advocacy' and 'linkage')
- Monitoring and evaluation
- Counselling (task centred, in the 'here and now')
- Graduated disengagement

Figure 3.6 Functions of the strengths model.

The functions are widely discussed in the literature (Kisthardt and Rapp, 1989; Kisthardt, 1992; Morgan, 1993) and many of them will be familiar from wider professional training. For the purposes of this text I wish to focus on specific relationship-orientated functions.

Engagement

In this particular model, engagement of the working relationship between client and case manager is seen as constituting a separate and distinct function in itself (Kisthardt and Rapp, 1989). This contrasts sharply with the majority of professional approaches that claim to consider the importance of the relationship, but in reality note 'assessment' as the first function of the process.

Engagement is seen as a series of unstructured, informal and shared encounters that take place at the beginning of the process of relationship building. Methods of engagement will be discussed in more detail in Chapter 5. Its purpose is inextricably linked to the central focus of the model, the need to establish a trusting individual relationship on which all other aspects of the work can be built.

By investing time and effort in developing trust and sharing information, we may be more certain that the move on to the specific strengths assessment will provide a more collaborative and complete assessment of strengths, wants, desires and aspirations. The more formalized approach of many professionals who aim to commence assessment of problems from the initial meetings tends to result in a more biased, professional-orientated assessment of the situation. Surely, they cannot claim comprehensiveness if the client has not been fully and equally engaged in the process.

A further value of the strengths model emphasis on initial engagement is the consideration it gives to the time required by many clients to accept and understand the case manager and the case management process. It should be remembered that meeting with a comparative stranger, at home or at a service base, and suddenly beginning to divulge your abilities and disabilities, your desires and fears is a rather unnatural situation. People in this client group have generally been through the problems-orientated assessments several times before, with a host of strangers, with little ultimate benefit to themselves. So, one aspect that may alleviate natural suspicion and achieve some appreciation would be a little more time and less pressure.

Graduated disengagement

At the opposite end of the helping relationship from engagement, the strengths model again deviates from the norm of traditional psychiatric practices. Rather than the sudden process of discharge from a service, the model presents the concept of graduated disengagement as a description of the reducing need for the services of intensive case management. The idea of termination representing a situation of the client doing well can have a negative effect, operating as a disincentive to get well if that means the loss of something that is clearly valued (Kisthardt and Rapp, 1989).

> Graduated disengagement ... is designed to increase contact with other providers and naturally occurring helpers in the community. ... This function is designed to prevent total dependence on the case

manager and to promote consumer empowerment, personal decision-making and autonomy ...

(*Kisthardt, 1992*)

The nature of the life experiences of this client group suggests that the relationship will be a long-term need, so no time limit can be planned for commencing the function of disengagement. It is envisaged that the timing is more likely to occur as a natural consequence of achieving goals and the changing nature of the relationship. However, as in all working relationships, the potential negative effects of dependency should be constantly monitored and addressed through a process of regular reviews.

Assessment and care planning

Within the strengths model of case management a subtle distinction can be drawn between the functions of assessing the client's 'wants', leading onto a planning of the 'needs' required in order to achieve these desires. In line with the overall philosophy of stressing motivation through a focus on the positive aspects of the individual, this model has drawn up specific documentation for recording the assessment of strengths and the planning of goal achievement (Kisthardt, 1992; Morgan, 1993). The strengths assessment is designed as a method of collecting information about the whole range of past achievements, current resources and future desires. It functions as a positive inventory when reflected back to the client, but stands alongside other professional assessments to supplement rather than replace existing information-gathering tools.

The specific focus on strengths and wants may occasionally draw criticisms of ignoring the very severe and disabling problems experienced by people in this client group, more so when the strengths approach denies the simplistic explanations that it is a mere positive reframing of identified problems. A major prerequisite of this approach is the humanitarian concern for the individual. The physical and psychological well-being of the client always remains paramount, so there is no denying that emergency precautions and formal detention procedures will be seen as necessary on occasions. What this approach stipulates is that the problems are usually reasonably obvious and as such, do not need the reinforcement that the special attention of assessment and care planning methods can present back to the client. In many circumstances the client will wish to express their perception of the problems and in fact may gain some inherent relief from so doing. This position would be accepted and encouraged within the framework of a strengths approach, but the predominant concern will be to help the client tackle the often more difficult expression of the positive aspects of their being.

In reality, some problems may frequently be resolved as a secondary effect of focusing on the achievement of goals towards longer term desires. Consideration of personal hygiene is a useful illustration; direct targeting of this daily activity through a problem-solving approach often fails because the individual is offered little or no tangible reward as a motivating force. From the strengths perspective, the focus of attention is directed constantly towards the achievement of a client's stated desire and the addressing of personal hygiene may become a spontaneous action if it is perceived by the client through the planning of goals to be a likely barrier to achieving what is desired.

This secondary resolution of problems is seen on a larger scale with the previous case study of Mehmet. For many years he has been the recipient of coercive services targeting medication compliance as the all-important goal, with repeated serious failures. Since the establishment of a case management presence, the discussion of medication and symptomatology has been a very frequent topic, but usually at the request of Mehmet himself. The case manager has chosen to help Mehmet focus more on his own desires of adequate housing, improving English literacy and sustaining a close personal relationship with a newfound partner. Mehmet sees his medication as one of the vital elements for helping him to achieve these goals.

SUMMARY

Case management is a comparatively recent organizational and clinical development in the provision of community services for people experiencing severe and long-term mental health problems. It has become the subject of intense scrutiny and discussion, with resulting claims to be an important element, but one which suffers from a lack of consensus about what it is or how it should be performed (Kanter, 1989).

The coordinating functions of a 'brokerage' model and the clinical functions of an 'intensive' model each have their place. The flexibility offered by such a range of services has contributed to the stability that case management can reflect to the client, which the more fragmented system of traditional psychiatric services has failed to do for the more needy client groups (Harris and Bergman, 1987).

In terms of service user and service provider relationships, the intensive models of case management have offered a new and effective method of working, but necessarily offering a comprehensive and long-term service. The strengths model offers a clear operational system, based on stated principles and a philosophy that upholds the relationship factor as essential to client outcomes, but at a necessary cost of low case load sizes (Rapp, 1988).

REFERENCES

Audit Commission (1986) *Making a Reality of Community Care*, HMSO, London.

Bachrach, L.L. (1989) Case management: toward a shared definition. *Hospital and Community Psychiatry*, **40**(9), 883–4.

Bachrach, L.L. (1992) The chronic patient: case management revisited. *Hospital and Community Psychiatry*, **43**(3), 209–10.

Brandon, D. and Towe, N. (1989) *Free to Choose: An Introduction to Service Brokerage*. Good Impressions Publishing, London.

Deitchman, W.S. (1980) How many case managers does it take to screw in a light bulb? *Hospital and Community Psychiatry*, **31**(11), 788–9.

DOH (1989) *Caring for People in the Next Decade and Beyond* (Cmnd 849), HMSO, London.

Goering, P.N., Wasylenki, D.A., Farkes, M., Lance, W. and Ballantyne, R. (1988) What difference does case management make? *Hospital and Community Psychiatry*, **39**(3), 272–6.

Griffiths, R. (1988) *Community Care: An Agenda for Action*, HMSO, London.

Harris, M. and Bergman, H.C. (1987) Case management with the chronically mentally ill: a clinical perspective. *American Journal of Orthopsychiatry*, **57**(2), 296–302.

Harris, M. and Bergman, H.C. (1988a) Clinical case management for the chronically mentally ill: a conceptual analysis. *New Directions for Mental Health Services*, **40**, 5–13.

Harris, M. and Bergman, H.C. (1988b) Misconceptions about the use of case management services by the chronically mentally ill: a utilization analysis. *Hospital and Community Psychiatry*, **39**(12), 1276–80.

Intagliata, J. (1982) Improving the quality of community care for the chronically mentally disabled: the role of case management. *Schizophrenia Bulletin*, **8**, 655–74.

Kanter, J. (1988) Clinical issues in the case management relationship, in *Clinical Case Management*, (eds M. Harris and L.L. Bachrach), Jossey-Bass, San Francisco.

Kanter, J. (1989) Clinical case management: definition, principles, components. *Hospital and Community Psychiatry*, **40**(4), 361–8.

Kisthardt, W.E. (1992) The strengths model of case management: the principles and functions of a helping partnership with persons with persistent mental illness, in *A Strengths Perspective for Social Work Practice*, (ed. D. Saleeby), Longman, New York pp. 59–83.

Kisthardt, W.E. and Rapp, C.A. (1989) *Bridging the Gap Between Principles and Practice: Implementing a Strengths Perspective in Case Management*, University of Kansas, Lawrence.

Morgan, S. (1993) *Community Mental Health: Practical Approaches to Long-term Problems*, Chapman & Hall, London.

NHS and Community Care Act (1990), HMSO, London.

Onyett, S. (1992) *Case Management in Mental Health*, Chapman & Hall, London.

Ovretveit, J. (1992) Concepts of case management. *British Journal of Occupational Therapy*, **55**(6), 225–8.

Prance, N. (1993) Travelling companions. *Nursing Times*, **89**(5), 28–30.

Rapp, C.A. (1988) *The Strengths Perspective of Case Management with Persons Suffering from Severe Mental Illness*, NIMH and University of Kansas, Lawrence.

Rapp, C.A. and Kisthardt, W.E. (1991) RDP Pilot Case Management Project. Workshop on the Strengths Model. Hoddesdon, November.

Rapp, C.A. and Wintersteen, R. (1989) The strengths model of case management: results from twelve demonstrations. *Psychological Rehabilitation Journal*, **13**(1), 23–32.

Repper, J. and Peacham, W. (1991) A suitable case for management? *Nursing Times*, **87**(12), 62–5.

Ryan, P., Ford, R. and Clifford, P. (1991) *Case Management and Community Care*, Research and Development for Psychiatry, London.

Sainsbury Centre for Mental Health (1994) Conference on 'Providing the Safety Net'. Imperial College, London.

Stein, L.I. and Test. M.A. (1980) Alternatives to mental hospital treatment. *Archives of General Psychiatry*, **37**, 392–7.

Weick, A., Rapp, C.A., Sullivan, W.P. and Kisthardt, W.E. (1989) A strengths perspective for social work practice. *Social Work*, **33**, 350–4.

Witheridge, T.F. (1989) The assertive community treatment worker: an emerging role and its implications for professional training. *Hospital and Community Psychiatry*, **40**(6), 620–4.

FURTHER READING

Ford, R., Beadsmore, A., Ryan, P. *et al.* (1995) Providing the safety net: case management for people with a serious illness. *Journal of Mental Health*, **1**, 91–7.

Franklin, J.L. (1988) Case management: a dissenting view. *Hospital and Community Psychiatry*, **39**(9), 921.

Harris, M. and Bergman, H. (eds) (1993) *Case Management for Mentally Ill Patients: Theory and Practice*, Langhorne, Harwood.

Shepherd, G. (1990) Case management. *Health Trends*, **22**(2), 59–61.

4

Therapeutic relationships

Before we consider the term 'therapeutic' in the structure of this text we need to more clearly identify the much broader notion of 'helping'. 'Helper skills' or 'helping relationships' are terms used by some writers as a means to de-emphasize the commonly held distinctions between the approach of the trained professional and that of the non-professional. Equal respect is attributed to the formalized models of helping adopted by the professional, to the volunteer counsellor and to the informal social support offered by family, friends or other carers (Wills, 1982; Nelson-Jones, 1988).

It may seem easy to conclude that we expect superior results from the investment in specialized training and a formalized process. There is no shortage of evidence to support the effectiveness of a wide range of therapies for clients (Smith *et al.*, 1980), as a review of any number of professional journals will testify. However, there are also studies to suggest very little difference in the overall effectiveness of highly trained professionals compared with the committed but untrained layperson (Durlak, 1979).

Wills (1982) suggests that by adopting the broader understanding of helping skills we enable an examination beyond that of pure skills, leading to '... a greater emphasis on situational factors in helping relationships and the effect that the context of the relationship has on the interaction between the participants'. One of the main themes of this text reflects this statement by suggesting that the specific client group respond as much, and possibly more, to the situation and context of the helping relationship as they do to the practice of specialized skills.

DEFINING AND REFINING 'THERAPEUTIC'

Most simple dictionary definitions link the concept to the activity of therapy, with grand allusions to healing, remedy and cure. In relation to this client group and the practice of psychiatry these terms raise quite inappropriate expectations and serve little real purpose, though it may be reasonably argued that 'remedial' actions are realistic methods of achieving some goals of therapy, e.g. participating in team-based sporting activity as a method of promoting fitness, self-awareness, concentration, social interaction, assertive behaviours, achievement. ...

For our purpose, 'therapeutic' relates more to the formalization of the method and process adopted by professionals as a direct result of their training, the conscious linking of planned goals to assessed needs through the medium of treatment. The term relates much less to the actual outcomes of the process. This ownership of terminology by the professional is highlighted further when we consider the practical reality of the informal carer, who is generally more free of the baggage of jargon. Family, friends and other informal carers are much more likely to use the terms 'help' or 'support', if pressed to describe what they do for a person; they are very unlikely to describe their own activity as being 'therapeutic'.

Consequently, we are able to narrow down the use of the term to the distinctive clinical approaches adopted by professionals for the purpose of developing interpersonal relationships through their different models of practice.

In essence, the therapeutic relationship which most professionals are striving to achieve may be distinguished by a number of characteristics:

- unilateral, with a focus on solving the problems of the client;
- formal, in its organization in time and place;
- time limited, in terms of the duration being defined by the achievement of stated goals and objectives;
- explicit or implicit contracts to guide behaviours within the boundaries of the relationship;
- approaches defined by stated models of professional practice;
- a narrow definition of the relationship, uncluttered by additional roles of friend, partner, parent.

These factors are clearly different from an informal helper role (Kanfer and Goldstein, 1986).

Therapeutic alliance

Whilst being broadly used by health professionals, this particular term is often preferred by medical practitioners to describe their relationship with a patient.

The purpose of such a therapeutic alliance is predominantly to facilitate compliance with prescribed medical treatments. There is no doubting the medical profession's appreciation of the need for some form of

relationship to be established, even to the extent of the frequent collo-
quial references to the quality of a doctor's 'bedside manner', However,
the nature of these relationships is arguably defined by the protocol of the
expert consultation based on a narrow appreciation of expert knowledge
and a strictly defined imbalance of power. In such circumstances, it may
be argued that the term 'therapeutic' is being somewhat hijacked to gloss
over the realities of the relationship, which largely depend on an unques-
tioned trust in the expertise of the medical professional.

Johnstone (1989), in reference to the practice of psychiatrists, suggests:

> ... modern medicine values the scientific rather than the empathic
> approach, i.e. diagnosis and the prescribing of physical treatments
> rather than counselling and an understanding of psychological
> factors ... such psychotherapeutic input as there is tends to be of
> little practical use in day-to-day patient management ...

The implications of these suggestions highlight contrasting roles in the
traditional doctor-patient relationship, whereby the medical practitioner
is in possession of the expertise and assumes responsibility for diagnosis,
treatment and prognosis while the patient assumes a more passive role of
trust (Parsons, 1951; Nelson-Jones, 1988).

Holistic

Nelson-Jones (1988) implies that the therapeutic approach is more holistic than that of the medical model described above.

A therapeutic approach requires the recipient to be an active participant who needs to work to maintain and develop the gains available from
therapy. They need to take on personal responsibility for positive change,
as the focus of the therapeutic interventions is to help people to make
changes for themselves.

Through the contrast of the medical and therapeutic approaches we
can begin to refine the latter more in terms of a relationship that focuses
on the potential for behavioural and emotional changes in the client. The
model of practice and the negotiable goals pursued by the professional
serve to distinguish an approach to relationships that actively promotes
the pursuit of change, rather than the treatment and relief of symptoms
of illness.

Therapeutic groupwork

The primary focus of this text is on the initiating and sustaining of relationships with people experiencing long-term severe distress, on an
individual basis. However, it is important to acknowledge in our review of
'therapeutic' interventions that a substantial amount of quite specialized

work takes place through the medium of therapeutic groups. Groupwork is seen as complementary to the individual therapeutic interventions, with a wide range of specific treatment aims and purposes. However, the necessary appreciation of the whole structure, function and management of therapeutic groups, leading to a study of group dynamics, would only serve to detract attention away from the focus of this text. I would refer the reader to other sources that give full and specialized attention to the subject of groupwork (Whittaker, 1985; Finlay, 1993).

PSYCHOTHERAPY AND COUNSELLING

A literal progression from the terms 'therapy' and 'therapeutic' would be a consideration of 'psychotherapy' and 'psychotherapeutic'.

Johnstone (1989) describes psychotherapy as the process of helping a person to understand and overcome their problems by encouraging them to talk through their life experiences in regular sessions with a trained psychotherapist. This is a very general definition and there are many different forms of psychotherapy depending on training, models of practice and theoretical frameworks.

Our particular client group and the models of psychotherapy share a somewhat chequered relationship. Primarily the client group is superficially excluded from psychotherapeutic interventions as a result of generalizations regarding interpersonal difficulties, psychotic symptoms which distort perceptions, poor insight into the condition, difficulties with all aspects of communication and a potential to be negatively stimulated by the cognitive demands of psychotherapy. As a defence for such exclusion criteria it is suggested that '... in the psychotherapeutic relationship clients are typically more active participants, in that they are likely to do more talking and initiate more topics of conversation during the session ...' (Schorr and Rodin, 1982).

Johnstone (1989) criticizes the approaches of psychotherapy for focusing almost solely on YAVIS (young, attractive, verbal, intelligent, successful) clients, to the exclusion of most people not of the same class or kind as the practising therapists. She suggests that the clients for whom we are concerned in this text are likely to be excluded from the verbal therapies and have to continue with the limited range of physical treatments offered by the medical profession.

Some redress of these pessimistic conclusions can be gained from the development of an annual Standing Conference on Psychotherapy of Schizophrenia in the UK since the early 1980s. There have also been a number of reviews published on the psychotherapeutic approaches to schizophrenia (Rogers, 1967; Wasylenki, 1992). Further developments of case management services for people with long-term mental health problems have also emphasized that the relationship encompasses all of the interpersonal dynamics inherent in psychotherapy (Kanter, 1988, 1989; Harris and Bergman, 1987).

In a simplistic view Johnstone (1989) suggests that counselling is essentially the same process as psychotherapy, practised in a more low-key way. This may point to a direction that holds more relevance to the needs of this client group.

In its pure form, counselling is defined as possessing the distinctive qualities of process, self-help, personal choices, a repertoire of skills, a relationship base and a focus on problems of living (Nelson-Jones, 1988). In this latter characteristic, it may illustrate its greater relevance to our client group through an emphasis on the practical here and now, whereas psychotherapy tends to focus much more on the personal historical and developmental experiences.

Burnard (1989) suggests that counselling is a practical activity, practised by many different people in many different ways. He describes it as an 'idiosyncratic mixture of personal qualities, practical skills and interpersonal verbal and non-verbal behaviours' that help a person to clarify and decide their own choices for action. The relationship is believed to belong to the client not the counsellor and the process is envisaged as a method of determining what the client wants rather than as a method of presenting the counsellor's repertoire of skills.

'Use of counselling skills'

For many people in the client group the notions of process and timescale linked to the tackling of problems seem less relevant than the immediate practical concerns of living with the disabilities of an unintelligible illness. With these circumstances in mind Kanter (1988) suggests that case management attempts to establish a collaborative relationship that addresses both the psychic and the environmental needs of the client. However, where the notions of process and timescale take a lower priority, the British Association of Counselling (1990) makes a clear distinction that this is not counselling in the professional sense of the term but might be described as 'use of counselling skills', which may be legitimately adopted by a range of professionals and volunteers as one aspect of their wide therapeutic interventions. However, because of the multiple roles that have to be performed, these people are less able to abide by the more formal contractual obligations that may be associated with pure counselling (Bayne and Nicolson, 1993). In practice, this loosening of contracts does not undermine the meeting of client needs; on the contrary, it more successfully achieves this aim for some clients who are discouraged by formality.

The relevance of therapeutic relationships with people in the client group becomes a little clearer when we consider the use of therapeutic skills in particular situations as a means for initiating and sustaining a relationship. This appears to be a more relevant reflection of need than the more formal process referred to earlier, though even the formal approaches should not be denied to someone on the basis of diagnosis, disability and duration, if they demonstrate a need and a potential to benefit from the application or even modification of such an approach.

With reference to the more loosely applied 'use of counselling skills', Johnstone (1989) highlights the value of simple human warmth that is frequently demonstrated in clinical settings by non-clinical staff such as administrative staff and domestic staff. She infers that the technicalities of professional training can often be detrimental to the practising of some of the simple natural helping instincts possessed by many people. These sentiments are further echoed by Nelson-Jones (1988) who suggests that ' ... helping skills are much too serious and valuable a thing to be left to professional helpers ...' Burnard (1989) advises us that we should not become too clever about our assumptions on how professional help can affect the lives of others; there should be no mystique about these skills as to varying degrees they are possessed and used by us all. However, at times the skills may even be misused, e.g. adopting patronizing tones towards a needy client.

Contracts, boundaries and limits

This is a further area of practice that arouses debate between those who present counselling as a formal process and those who use counselling skills as one part of a wider repertoire of interventions with clients. The implication is that a degree of role conflict may occur for people loosely using counselling skills if they attempt to formalize the negotiation of boundaries and contracts. Arguably the 'process' view takes a rather limited and somewhat possessive stance on the use of these formal procedures. As with the case of using skills, so the use of formal procedures may be adapted to more specific circumstances.

A contract is a formal explicit agreement which helps to ensure the professional nature of the relationship (Stewart, 1992). It is agreed between a 'counsellor' and a 'client' at the outset of the relationship and helps to define the purpose and approach of the therapeutic intervention, as well as outlining the practical arrangements and conditions of the work to be undertaken (Bayne et al., 1994). It may be formal or informal, verbal or written. A contract may be used as a positive definition of the therapeutic relationship but it may also be used as a negative or punitive measure for restricting or compelling a client's behaviour.

Case study 4.1: Burt (51 years old)

Experiences a diagnosis of schizophrenia, with persistent delusional ideas that his face is changing to resemble an animal. Disabled by obsessional thought patterns and behaviours, with feelings of tension and weakness throughout his body. Burt becomes socially isolated and withdrawn, with periods of increasing dependency on his family and on the taking of sleeping tablets.

The nature of the positive application of a contract with Burt took the form of using a community team information sheet. Whilst this sheet only gave general statements about the service and contact numbers, Burt and the case manager discussed the priorities of service need and put them in writing on the back of the sheet. Adding names and places to the offers of service personalized the information in a form of an agreement with Burt.

Case study 4.2: Anna (27 years old)

Experiences a diagnosis of schizophrenia, complicated by frequent drug abuse. Holds major concerns about her own sexuality which can lead her to make dramatic changes to her appearance through shaving her head, using strongly masculine clothing and adopting male names. Funds her drug abuse through prostitution; can become aggressive and threatening towards others through racist taunts and gestures. Occasionally arrested for threatening use of knives, re-entering psychiatric services through the legal system.

At times a more restrictive use of contracts needs to be negotiated with Anna. She will be asked to hand over any offensive weapons before being seen by workers. She is given strict appointment times to ensure that the same workers can see her; she is not allowed access to the building at other times and is reminded of the specific appointment times. Contracts in these circumstances are needed to give Anna some consistency, and to promote levels of safety for all people involved.

One aspect of a contract may be the defining of appropriate boundaries for the therapeutic relationship. This enables the relationship to be set in clear and trusting limits that create the necessary stability for working on stated objectives (Bayne et al., 1994). Relevant boundaries would include timing, duration, location, structure and confidentiality within the relationship.

Case study 4.3: Tony (39 years old)

Experiences a diagnosis of schizophrenia, with a forensic history detailing numerous petty criminal offences and one serious incident of assault causing grievous bodily harm in response to instructions from hallucinatory voices. Tony presents mainly as quiet and withdrawn, abuses alcohol to a mild degree which further aggravates physical problems such as stomach ulcers. He continues to hold angry feelings towards one previous acquaintance.

Much of the supportive relationship with Tony focuses on the practical issues of housing, finance and work skills training. He reports significant positive changes in many aspects of his life, but no change in very specific feelings of anger. A contract was drawn up to establish a specific therapeutic relationship through which Tony may use a counselling approach to discussing this particular difficulty. The contract specified the number of sessions, time, duration and place. It was decided to hold these sessions in a separate location from the more usual meetings to plan and discuss other practical tasks. This would help Tony to focus his attention more specifically on the reasons for counselling by providing the external stimuli of a changed environment. Thus the boundaries were tightly defined for a specific type of therapeutic relationship. This approach was felt to be particularly helpful in Tony's circumstances.

It is reasonably easy to understand how the drawing of boundaries can help to define the professional nature of a formal counselling process. However, in the experiences of case management services there is the constant temptation to slip into ambiguity as a result of drifting from the professional relationship into that of friendship. The very practical nature of the interventions, combined with the comprehensive areas of assessment and support, makes it easy to fall into the trap of such ambiguity. In these situations it becomes vitally important that the case manager is constantly examining the boundaries and the limits of changing and developing relationships. Furthermore, it can be an essential part of the therapeutic nature of the interventions to be constantly discussing these boundaries and limits with the client. If we identify interpersonal relationships as being a frequent area of difficulty for people, then the very nature of discussing and highlighting boundaries and limits should act as an intervention targeted to a specific need.

The setting of boundaries becomes less formalized in the situations of informally 'using counselling skills', rather than the more formal 'counselling process'. However, there is the frequent danger of careless boundaries leading to the greater ambivalence mentioned above, with a lesser clarity about the function of the therapeutic relationship.

We need to communicate clearly what can be expected of a person as a professional and as a human being, though it needs to be quite obvious that the human aspect does not stray into the personal, sexual or family friend roles. Behaviours that may be acceptable at a close personal level are not appropriate at a professional therapeutic level. Similarly, expectations that an individual professional can be contacted at any time, day or night, are not necessarily helpful to the development of an effective therapeutic relationship. Boundaries on time availability may also helpfully specify other individuals or other services that are accessible for other times of the day or week.

The boundaries and the limits can be set by a process of negotiation between the client and the professional. Further limitations may be set on the therapeutic relationship by a host of other factors:

• the skill of the therapist;
• the willingness of a client to engage in the relationship;
• different expectations of the outcome between the client and the therapist;
• the policies and priorities of the employing agency;
• the location of interactions, e.g. office, street, client's home;
• the influence of other people, e.g. informal carers.

THE 'SKILLS' AND 'RELATIONSHIP' DEBATE

The psychiatrist Jerome D. Frank has suggested that the interpersonal relationship between helper and client is the primary ingredient of therapeutic change, regardless of the type of therapy employed (Di Nicola and Di Matteo, 1982). However, when considering the volume of studies into the nature of the one-to-one relationship the debate still continues about which elements of the therapeutic process are responsible for change: 'acquired skills' or 'natural relationship factors' (Wills, 1982). Lloyd and Maas (1991) suggest that caring alone is not sufficient and that the relationship cannot function independently of the attitudes, values and skills brought by the therapist.

Whilst some people may be motivated to change and will thus enter into a therapeutic relationship with positive expectations, others are more resistant for reasons of mistrust, anger, fear of possible symptoms of illness, such as a formal thought disorder that distorts the more natural perceptions of interpersonal contacts. It may be assumed that the motivated person will achieve some positive effect of basic human warmth and respect from the relationship itself, whereas the resistant individual may require the therapist to apply specific skills in order to win over their trust and cooperation.

Much of the remainder of this chapter will examine skills factors and relationship factors separately, but we should always appreciate and understand the close interconnection between them. It is the use of particular skills that will help to engender the relationship, as well as the therapeutic outcomes. Similarly, it is the security offered by the boundaries of the relationship that enables attention to focus on the skills employed to help achieve the agreed therapeutic goals.

INTERPERSONAL SKILLS

An essential element of any effective therapeutic approach is self-awareness:

> ... the gradual and continuous process of noticing and exploring aspects of the self, whether behavioural, psychological or physical, with the intention of developing personal and interpersonal understanding. Such awareness ... is intimately bound up with our relationships with others. To become more aware of and to have a deeper understanding of ourselves is to have a sharper and clearer picture of what is happening to others.
>
> *(Burnard, 1992)*

Self-awareness enables us to make conscious decisions about our choice of words and practice of counselling skills. It enables us to separate out what psychological material belongs to us and what belongs to the client, stopping any overidentification with the client's problems or projecting our own onto the client.

When considering the wide range of available counselling skills, it may be helpful to adopt a broader categorization:

1. **Initiative skills**: involve the therapist being proactive, establishing an initial rapport or contact by putting the client at ease with the therapist and the proposed therapeutic interventions.
2. **Facilitative skills**: involve the therapist being proactive, helping to develop the client's understanding, probing for deeper understanding, further information or alternative perspectives.
3. **Responsive skills**: involve the therapist being reactive, responding to the thoughts, behaviours and actions of the client, leading to further facilitated understanding.

The counselling skills listed in Table 4.1 are grouped simply under these three categories. Many would appear in more than one category, but for simplicity are only listed in what is considered to be their primary function.

Lloyd and Maas (1991, 1992) suggest that for a relationship to be truly therapeutic the core helper dimensions of empathy, respect, genuineness and concreteness need to be present in high degrees. Other writers, whilst stressing the central importance of empathy, point specifically to listening and attending as the most in. ortant of the counselling skills (Burnard, 1989, 1992).

Table 4.1 Categories of counselling skills

Initiative	Facilitative	Response
Acceptance	Accenting	Clarification
Attending	Challenging	Concreteness
Empathy	Confronting	Feedback
Genuineness	Humour	Focusing
Listening	Immediacy	Interpretation
Openness	Intuition	Paraphrasing
Respect	Minimal prompts	Reassurance
Trust	Questioning	Reflection
Warmth	Structuring	Reframing
		Self-disclosure
		Silence
		Summarizing
		Touch

Empathy

Empathy is a skill most central to counselling and all other forms of therapy. It is an ability to enter the world of another person and experience that world through their frame of reference with no prejudgements from your own perspective. Put more simply, it is the ability to see the world through someone else's eyes.

Empathy is about understanding the thoughts and feelings of another person through their own personal meaning. Moreover, empathic understanding can only truly take place when the therapist has communicated meaning back to the client. It is not to be misinterpreted as sympathy or pity for another person. Stewart (1992) makes the following simple distinctions:

> Empathy is to feel 'with',
> Sympathy is to be 'like'
> Pity is to feel 'for'.

Empathy may be fleetingly used to great value with a person who presents as seriously thought disordered with severely disturbed experiences. A most typical response is to contain and physically treat the symptoms, without necessarily acknowledging the reality of the experiences to the person themselves. When prioritizing the need to stabilize the disturbing effects as quickly as possible, the additional benefit of a therapeutic relationship may be denied in these circumstances. However, the use of empathic responses that acknowledge the reality, the pain and even the horror of such experiences may present the additional support of a caring and understanding relationship at a time of severe emotional trauma.

Such empathic responses may help to initiate or maintain a therapeutic relationship at the time of most severe distress, which can then be built on or continued through the stabilizing and recovering period. Failure to use such an opportunity means a worker may need to initiate a relationship from a more disadvantageous position, with a client feeling additionally damaged by the powerlessness of a situation where they were aggressively treated without much concern for their specific feelings of distress.

Use of such interpersonal skills in times of distress and disturbance needs to be placed in the context of an assessment of risk, both in terms of the physical risk to client or staff resulting from the disturbing experiences and an assessment of how much the empathy reinforces the experience of disturbed behaviours. Thus, it may be a skill to be used fleetingly, to indicate an acknowledgement of what the client is communicating but then to place this experience alongside reality as it is being experienced by others.

Case study 4.4: Abdul (25 years old)

Experiencing a diagnosis of schizophrenia, Abdul had retreated to his bed 24 hours a day, refusing to have sheets on the bed because of a persistent preoccupation with sand and dust associated with his native Morocco.

In order to initiate a working relationship it was necessary for the case manager to engage in discussions about dust in Morocco and its potential discomforting sensations if the bedsheets were to become covered in dust and sand. By occasionally entering into Abdul's frame of reference the case manager was able to demonstrate a concern to share his experiences. This form of acknowledgement, demonstrated through a fleeting degree of empathy, enabled the initiation of a relationship that could then be tentatively used to explore other perceptions of Abdul's situation and behaviours.

The alternative approach of discounting Abdul's frame of reference bluntly as a symptom of illness requiring physical treatment failed to gain anything more than the negative responses of confrontation and threats of aggression interspersed with periods of non-communication with Abdul retreating beneath his duvet.

Empathy is described as the most central of the core conditions of the person-centred approach to therapeutic relationships outlined by the work of Carl Rogers (1951, 1967). It is determined as much by the communication of intuition as it is by any more tangible technical skill. However, Burnard (1989) warns us that levels of empathy can be limited by differences of culture, education and philosophy. Like all of the counselling skills, empathy is something possessed by all of us to different degrees and can be developed through practice.

Listening

Nelson-Jones (1988) suggests there is a clear distinction between hearing and listening, the latter involving an additional degree of understanding the full meaning of what is being said. We are not only concerned with the linguistic aspects of speech such as phrases and metaphors, but also with the paralinguistic aspects of tone, rate and volume. The meaning is also more accurately understood if we are also concerned with body language, where occasionally there may be significant incongruence between what is being communicated non-verbally and what is actually being said. Accurate listening enhances our ability to gain the trust of a client, thus establishing a sense of rapport. It also helps us to encourage the client to express some of their more deeper personal feelings, particularly if they perceive that they will be listened to without the recipient making quick judgements.

People in this client group frequently feel they are not being listened to, whether by family or professional staff. Other people appear quick to pass judgement or make a diagnosis or imply that they have heard it all before because of a person's long history of illness. Many in this client group feel that others are only listening for what they expect to hear or for what will give clues to a diagnosis or relapse of the same condition.

Attending

This is the act of truly focusing our attention on the other person, consciously making ourselves aware of what they are trying to communicate to us. Lloyd and Maas (1992) suggest it is a way of helping the client to feel important, that their concerns and feelings are valued by the therapist. Attending can be enhanced by adopting a relaxed body posture, using physical openness, an occasional slight forward lean and good eye contact and by restricting other environmental distractions (Burnard, 1989, 1992).

Burnard (1989) outlines three levels of attention:

1. focus out – onto the client and environment;
2. focus in – onto our own thoughts and feelings engendered by what the client is communicating;
3. focus on fantasy – onto what you think may be happening rather than on what is actually being said.

All three levels play a part in enhancing our information about the client's circumstances, but we should concentrate our efforts on focusing out, with occasional checks of the other two levels.

Use of questions

A temptation that frequently presents itself in the effort to establish inter-personal communication is the need to ask the client questions. This may be particularly acute when confronted by the protracted silences of a withdrawn or fearful person or someone who is essentially resistant to the approaches of staff. Even the thought-disordered or very preoccupied person many engender a similar urge to overcompensate with a series of questions. Nelson-Jones (1988) expresses a major reservation about the use of questions in the therapeutic relationship, particularly if they have the effect of taking the client out of their frame of reference into that of the therapist or even into some unproductive neutral territory. He does acknowledge that the judicious use of questions may help the client to explore, clarify and understand their own frame of reference.

The skill lies in judging the timing and balance of questions. There are particular functions, such as the information gathering of assessment procedures, that require more attention to questions. Ideally the assessment would not begin until a degree of relationship building had been initiated, in order for it to be a more cooperative venture and hence more accurate.

Accepting that there will be times when a therapist will need to make use of questions, Nelson-Jones (1988) suggests we try to avoid using:

- too many questions, giving an impression of interrogation;
- leading questions, reducing the options to answer;
- closed questions that only demand a yes/no answer;
- over-elaborate and wordy questions;
- poor timing that interrupts the flow or raises negative reactions;
- 'why' questions, which seem like an interrogation.

It may help to use questions that offer the client opportunities to explore further meaning, deeper feeling or more specific understanding (Dillon, 1990). The most sensitive method would be to use few questions, short questions and open questions, e.g.:

What do you think will happen?
How did that make you feel?
What do you think you might do?

Self-disclosure

Allied to the therapist's use of questions, in a proactive sense, is the use of self-disclosure: 'The process by which we let ourselves be known to others' (Stewart, 1992). Nelson-Jones (1988) outlines a number of reasons why we may wish to use this skill:

- a method of demonstrating the therapeutic process to a client;
- appearing genuine and involved;
- sharing personal experiences common to both people;
- provide feedback to help client's understanding of their own experience.

However, there are potential dangers when using this skill in the therapeutic relationship:

- unintentionally burdening client with our own problems;
- can appear weak and unstable if you are presenting yourself as a person with multiple difficulties;
- dominating the relationship through the therapist's possession of communication.

Used sensitively, self-disclosure can be a constructive response within a developing therapeutic relationship (Lloyd and Maas, 1992). However, it is a skill that needs to be used cautiously and Nelson-Jones (1988) offers the following guidelines:

- Be self-referent, rather than using third party experiences.
- Be to the point.
- Be sensitive to the client's needs.
- Do not overuse this skill.

Use of humour

At a superficial level, humour may appear to be an inappropriate or contradictory therapeutic response, particularly with people who have serious, painful and disabling experiences of prolonged mental health problems. Stewart (1992) suggests that we should distinguish between humour that is used to attack and humour that is used as a shared response. An example of attacking humour would be the therapist focusing on the client's disability with a malicious intent to highlight the inequality of power between them. This would not only be inappropriate but potentially very damaging to a therapeutic relationship. Bayne *et al.* (1994) suggest that humour can be useful in offering new perspectives, e.g. seeing the absurd aspect of circumstances can help to gain some control by alleviating a sense of hopelessness.

The appropriate use of humour in the therapeutic relationship can potentially:

- lower anxiety, stress and even aggression;
- reduce the emotional distance between client and therapist;
- focus attention on specific material;
- assist in developing the relationship.

It needs to be well timed and intentionally focused in a specific direction. It would be improper to advocate the reduction of therapeutic interventions to pure comedy, but the ability to share even a brief smile at some humourous aside can greatly benefit the relationship. For people who are more used to the serious aspects of their difficulties, it can be quite refreshing for somebody to adopt a lighter attitude towards their circumstances. However, inappropriately used humour can have a disastrous effect on the relationship, so it is better to be well informed about an individual client's circumstances or to make light of only very safe subjects, e.g. the government, Social Services or the hospital in general.

Unconditional positive regard

Interpersonal skills for inviting and facilitating a therapeutic relationship should always be employed in a manner that acknowledges and values the individual client, whoever they are and whatever their experiences may be. This notion reflects a central theme of Carl Rogers' approach to client-centred therapy, the very essence of the humanistic approach, which is unconditional positive regard. This phrase describes 'a non-possessive caring and acceptance of the client, irrespective of how offensive their behaviour might be ... we communicate a deep and genuine caring, not filtered through our own feelings, thoughts, and behaviours ... (Stewart, 1992).

By assuming a positive attitude towards a client, we enable them to more easily enter into a therapeutic relationship, through which they may subsequently be able to evaluate and reappraise some of their own values and behaviours. Any initial rejection of their values and behaviours makes a therapeutic relationship all the more difficult to initiate, as the starting point would be more likely to focus on incongruence and confrontation. The potential for facilitating evaluation and positive change would then be much more difficult to achieve.

INTERPERSONAL RELATIONSHIP FACTORS

Nelson-Jones (1988) suggests that the development of a therapeutic relationship involves a great deal of risk, particularly as the client may perceive that they will have to reveal a great deal of very personal information. Whilst effective counselling skills can be employed to support and contain the level of risk, there are also inherent factors in the relationship itself which may enhance or detract from this very outcome. Fisher and Nadler (1982) outline what they consider to be donor, recipient and context characteristics which may intrinsically influence the development of the relationship between a client and a helper.

Primary among these characteristics is the client's perceptions of positive bonding with a particular therapist. This may result from similarities in physical appearance or from a less tangible feeling of the client being accepted and respected by the therapist.

The therapist's personality, ability and general attitude have been highlighted by Lloyd and Maas (1991) as aspects of the interpersonal relationship that may engender a more positive interaction. Bayne and Nicholson (1993) express this aspect in terms of the therapist respecting the client's values, attitudes and sense of self-determination, corresponding closely to the previous discussion of unconditional positive regard. If the client perceives the therapist to be someone who will make positive judgements and decisions, they may be more attracted into a therapeutic relationship.

Lloyd and Maas (1991) suggest that not all caring or helping relationships are therapeutic; at times the therapist may respond neither empathically nor effectively to the client. Fehrenbach and O'Leary (1982) outline how 'attributional bias' can influence the development of a relationship. This is where the therapist potentially or actually attributes the client's difficulties to aspects of their personality, whereas the client attributes any blame to situational or external factors. Such incongruence, whether real or perceived, can have a detrimental influence on the development of a therapeutic relationship.

Schorr and Rodin (1982) investigate the relationship in terms of perceived or actual control. They suggest that typically the client must relinquish some control in the therapeutic relationship because of the very nature of professional consultations and because they bring to the relationships problems or difficulties for resolution or change. However, the client's perception of how this control is used or abused by the therapist may have a significant bearing on the development of the relationship itself.

Much of the work outlined in this chapter presupposes that a relationship can be developed and nurtured over time, particularly with clients who are perceived to be resistant or difficult in some way. However, there is evidence to suggest that relationships can be initiated very quickly, based on some unquantifiable factors of mutual liking or through immediately establishing congruent ideas about the expectations of the therapeutic relationship and its potential outcomes. Lloyd and Maas (1992) suggest that the initial contact between therapist and client can be very significant in determining the nature and quality of the relationship that will develop between them. Wills (1982) points to evidence which suggests that the mutual attraction, upon which subsequent outcomes may be strongly determined, occurs within the first two or three meetings. Introducing yourself in a natural manner, asking the client what they want for the future and genuinely acknowledging the importance of going at the client's pace can together represent a change from the expected initial contact with professionals and set up the right kind of conditions for working together in many cases.

FURTHER PRACTICAL APPLICATIONS OF COUNSELLING SKILLS

The different varieties of counselling are far too numerous to cover at this point, but I will draw attention to a few broad categories that are frequently used with people in this client group. Some forms of counselling may need conscious decisions and preparation to be made by the therapist, acknowledging the value of the process and adapting degrees of formality to client need. Some forms of counselling are performed fleetingly, in response to immediate needs, often without conscious thought of the skills being used. It is these latter instances that I would wish to highlight as being more responsive to the need of the client group, but all too often devalued by the academic focus on higher level cognitive processes and procedures that venture into the realms of psychotherapy.

Supportive counselling

The most frequently used method of counselling, either as a planned intervention or more often as an immediate response to need. It takes the form of the therapist acting as a sounding board for the client's ideas, plans, suggestions, worries, fears or anxieties. The primary skills involved are those of listening and attending, with an additional level of empathic understanding which should be communicated clearly in response.

Case study 4.5: Richard (46 years old)

Experiencing a 22 year history of manic depressive psychosis, with frequent relapses, arrests, detention on sections of the Mental Health Act and treatment against his will. Richard showed an early ability to achieve in terms of work skills and other occupational endeavours, but the years in the psychiatric system have frustrated his desires and abilities, seriously impaired his relationships with others and filled him with a sense of anger and resentment.

A frequent role for the case manager is to give Richard the opportunity to vent his feelings of entrapment by the system and reflect back the sense of helplessness but to also acknowledge that he still has abilities and the potential to adapt to changing opportunities. The supportive counselling role can take the form of a planned joint visit off the hospital ward to a local café for a discussion or it can be a quite immediate need for release of tension on the ward when Richard perceives that hospital staff are not considering his views on the needs for treatment.

Informative counselling

Clients may frequently ask for specific information about their condition, illness or planned treatment. The sensitive response to such requests through the giving of information is what constitutes informative counselling. We are in effect fulfilling a vital obligation to help people make informed decisions and choices about their health and their treatment. Frequently, the giving of such information requires a counselling approach because of the sensitivity of the subject matter, because information is often claimed to be withheld from the client and because the information sometimes results in conflicting standpoints about the decisions that could be made, e.g. the accepting of depot injection medication while formally detained under the Mental Health Act.

Case study 4.6: Mehmet (35 years old)

Experiencing a long history of being diagnosed with schizophrenia. Many hospital admissions, formally detained, following assaults on other people, generally after actively stopping medication or occasionally by adding illegal drugs while still remaining on low doses of antipsychotic medications.

Mehmet had recently engaged in a personal relationship, which caused him to seriously examine his own actions over many years in the psychiatric system. Supportive counselling was a necessary element of his treatment during the periods of depressive contemplation over what he saw as a wasted life. With some degree of insight Mehmet began to ask staff serious questions about his psychiatric condition, the medication effects and the influence of illegal drugs on him. As a result Mehmet has been able to use informative counselling to make better informed choices about continuing his treatment, with an additional sense of being able to negotiate the levels of medication that he is prepared to accept. He also feels a need to know more about signs of relapse, in order to prevent a recurrence of the worst aspects of his history.

Occupational counselling

The experience of major mental health problems is widely accepted as having a serious effect on a person's access to work, study and wider leisure pursuits. Through the inevitable financial penalties of broken or terminated work income, access to other opportunities becomes diminished. Most people still express a desire to return to full-time productive employment, for social as well as financial reasons. The broader 'occupational' options of employment, volunteering, training, education and leisure may still offer a range of opportunities. The individual client facing decisions about their own future will frequently require some help and guidance to search out and evaluate the potential options.

Case study 4.7: Buki (51 years old)

A 26-year history diagnosed with schizophrenia has seriously interrupted the intellectual and occupational potential that Buki had when she initially arrived in England from Nigeria in the 1960s. Periods of mental health problems have rendered her catatonic in presentation, very slowed up and feeling weak and unable to cope with family responsibilities. Brief periods of unskilled manual work had previously triggered relapses of her condition.

Over a period of three years Buki and her case manager have frequently discussed and evaluated options for steadily increasing her levels of activity, but at a deliberately slow pace so as not to trigger relapses as previously. Through the use of informal drop-ins, formalized groupwork, limited access to her children in Social Services care and her contacts with a local church, Buki has steadily increased her involvement from half a day a week to five days a week of routine and structure. She is now considering an employment rehabilitation course, with realistic views towards part-time employment.

Counselling in emotional distress

This form can be planned if a client's history dictates such a frequent need, but more often takes the form of a sudden and unplanned response to immediate need. Once again the primary skills are those of listening, attending and empathy.

The full expression of feelings should be encouraged and often this release and someone to listen will suffice to relieve much of the distress.

Case study 4.8: Gayle (39 years old)

Following an early career in a healthcare profession, Gayle has experienced 12 years of disabling intractably deep depression, with frequent suicidal ideas and intent. Whilst she has brief periods of recovery and hope, she appears to plunge rapidly back into despair and hopelessness, without clearly identifiable causes.

For Gayle there is a need to plan the availability of supportive counselling, but also to make plans for the sudden and frequent episodes of intense emotional distress. Whilst on a hospital ward response can be rapid, the periods of time when Gayle is at home present a problem if suicidal ideas form rapidly. Help and encouragement to use telephone counselling are combined with attempts to respond with rapid home visits and with frequent planned visits by Gayle to the community team.

SUMMARY

The term 'therapeutic', when applied to the development of interpersonal relationships, refers to a professional focus on the need for process, models of practice and the linking of assessed needs to goals of achievement. At its most exact level we are referring to the approaches of psychotherapy and formal counselling, but in relation to a long-term client group the distinction of 'using counselling skills' is more relevant than the formal process (Bayne and Nicolson, 1993).

Essentially the use of counselling skills is a process of listening and talking with a client with the intention of helping them to come to decisions about what further actions they can take (Burnard, 1992). It is a very practical activity, accessible to all and not to be shrouded in any mystique (Burnard, 1989). Arguably it is less about what we do for others and more about what we help them to do for themselves (Nelson-Jones, 1988).

Much of the professional debate surrounds the relative importance for a therapeutic approach of acquired skills or intrinsic relationship factors. Burnard (1989) suggests that client-centred counselling evolves through the relationship itself, but that the practice of specific skills helps to give the process some shape. Lloyd and Maas (1991) argue that caring alone is not sufficient and that you need the skills as well as the values and attitudes of the therapist in order to achieve effective therapeutic outcomes.

The initiating and sustaining of therapeutic relationships will depend to varying extents on both the skills and the interpersonal factors. Perhaps the more important practical consideration is just how widely applicable therapeutic relationships are to people in this client group. Much work is done through the unplanned supportive counselling response to need, as well as the more formal planning of therapeutic goals. This fact should not be lost in the academic debate that frequently tends to apply therapeutic relationships more to the formal development of counselling and psychotherapy.

REFERENCES

Bayne, R. and Nicolson, P. (eds) (1993) *Counselling and Psychology for Health Professionals*, Chapman & Hall, London.

Bayne, R., Horton, I., Merry, T. and Noyes, E. (1994) *Counsellor's Handbook*, Chapman & Hall, London.

British Association of Counselling (1990) *Code of Ethics and Practice for Counsellors*, BAC, Rugby.

Burnard, P. (1989) *Counselling Skills for Health Professionals*, Chapman & Hall, London.

Burnard, P. (1992) *Effective Communication Skills for Health Professionals*, Chapman & Hall, London.

Dillon, J.T. (1990) *The Practice of Questioning*, Routledge, London.

Di Nicola, D.D. and Di Matteo, M.R. (1982) Communication, interpersonal influence and resistance to medical treatment, in *Basic Processes in Helping Relationships*, (ed. T.A.Wills), Academic Press, New York.

Durlak, J.A. (1979) Comparative effectiveness of paraprofessional and professional helpers. *Psychological Bulletin,* **86**, 80–92.

Fehrenbach, P.A. and O'Leary, M.R. (1982) Interpersonal attraction and treatment decisions in in-patient and out-patient psychiatric settings, in *Basic Processes in Helping Relationships*, (ed. T.A. Wills), Academic Press, New York.

Finlay, L. (1993) *Groupwork in Occupational Therapy*, Chapman & Hall, London.

Fisher, J.D. and Nadler, A. (1982) Determinants of recipient reactions to aid: donor–recipient similarity and perceived dimensions of problems, in *Basic Processes in Helping Relationships*, (ed. T.A.Wills), Academic Press, New York.

Harris, M. and Bergman, H.C. (1987) Case management with the chronically mentally ill: a clinical perspective. *American Journal of Orthopsychiatry,* **57**(2), 296–302.

Johnstone, L. (1989) *Users and Abusers of Psychiatry. A Critical Look at Traditional Psychiatric Practice,* Routledge, London.

Kanfer, F.H. and Goldstein, A.P. (eds) (1986) *Helping People Change*, 3rd edn, Pergamon Press, Oxford.

Kanter, J. (1988) Clinical issues in the case management relationship, in *Clinical Case Management*, (eds M. Harris and L.L. Bachrach), Jossey-Bass, San Francisco.

Kanter, J. (1989) Clinical case management: definition, principles, components. *Hospital and Community Psychiatry,* **40**(4), 361–8.

Lloyd, C. and Maas, F. (1991) The therapeutic relationship. *British Journal of Occupational Therapy,* **54**(3), 111–13.

Lloyd, C. and Maas, F. (1992) Interpersonal skills and occupational therapy. *British Journal of Occupational Therapy,* **55**(10), 379–82.

Nelson-Jones, R. (1988) *Practical Counselling and Helping Skills*, 2nd edn, Cassell, London.

Parsons, T. (1951) *The Social System*, Free Press, New York.

Rogers, C.R. (1951) *Client-Centred Therapy*, Constable, London.

Rogers, C.R. (1967) *On Becoming a Person: A Therapist's View of Psychotherapy*, Constable, London.

Schorr, D. and Rodin, J. (1982) The role of perceived control in practitioner–patient relationships, in *Basic Processes in Helping Relationships*, (ed. T.A. Wills), Academic Press, New York.

Smith, M.L., Glass, G.V. and Miller, T.I. (1980) *The Benefits of Psychotherapy*, Johns Hopkins University Press, Baltimore.

Stewart, W. (1992) *A–Z of Counselling Theory and Practice,* Chapman & Hall, London.

Wasylenki, D.A. (1992) Psychotherapy of schizophrenia revisited. *Hospital and Community Psychiatry*, **43**(2), 123–7.

Whittaker, D.S. (1985) *Using Groups to Help People*, Routledge and Kegan Paul, London.

Wills, T.A. (ed.) (1982) *Basic Processes in Helping Relationships*, Academic Press, New York.

FURTHER READING

Barrett-Lennard, G.T. (1981) The empathy cycle: refinement of a nuclear concept. *Journal of Counselling Psychology*, **28**, 91–100.

Bond, T. (1993) Counselling, counselling skills and professional roles, in *Counselling and Psychology for Health Professionals*, (eds R. Bayne and P. Nicolson), Chapman & Hall, London, pp. 3–14.

Ivey, A.E. (1987) *Counselling and Psychotherapy: Skills, Theories and Practice*, Prentice-Hall, London.

Murgatroyd, S. (1985) *Counselling and Helping*, Methuen, London.

Supportive relationships | 5

The focus of this chapter is placed clearly with the practical tasks of daily living and with attempts to maintain levels of social contact with people who are essentially very vulnerable. Some people are adversely affected by the changing organization of the social and political conditions that shape our lives. In terms of their mental health, they may well have adapted to circumstances by minimizing contact with other people, but their isolation does not completely protect them from the ever-changing circumstances around them. The sudden encroachment of change can greatly unsettle an otherwise stable degree of mental functioning, causing a possibly 'chronic' but settled mental state to suddenly become a serious cause for concern.

Alternatively, some people may experience a more actively chaotic and/or possibly volatile reaction to changes and social organization. Once again, losing a sense of control of the myriad influences and requirements made on our daily lives may cause a disturbance in the ability to function as fully and competently as society expects of us. The snowball effect results in adverse influences on the state of mental functioning, with further chaos or volatility as a defence against the increasing sense of pressure.

Consequently, the supportive relationship is about trying to initiate and maintain some form of contact with people who traditionally resist the approaches of helping agencies. For some, this resistance may be a result of quite real or perceived feelings that the psychiatric system is not responsive to their particular needs. The system can often be seen to focus on symptoms of illness and the need for treatment whereas for many if not most clients, the priorities are the basic human concerns of living in comfortable housing, with sufficient money to pay the bills and the type of social and occupational activity that suits them personally (Pilling,

1991). Their own experience of the system may frequently be one of coercion when these priorities are seen to be in conflict. In the extreme, this experience may involve 'sectioning' into hospital, under powers of the Mental Health Act (1983), even involving the presence of the police on occasions.

Resistance in this client group has all too often been met with unintentionally apathetic responses by the system. Finite and stretched resources are allocated according to service priorities and people who are seen as reluctant and in need of chasing do not figure so highly. Some people not surprisingly slip through the net, only to find themselves a priority for urgent attention and treatment when the inevitable crisis arises.

Therapeutic relationships can be linked to the professional approach within service priorities, whereas the supportive relationship will frequently seek to prioritize the practical tasks identified as important by the client. That is not to deny, however, that the supportive relationship may equally be concerned with matters of mental functioning and medical treatments, where appropriate. The therapeutic relationship stresses the importance of helping the client to make their own choices and decisions about how to act; similar aims would be shared by the supportive relationship focus, though there may be a greater degree of 'getting alongside and working with' the client. This may involve carrying out practical tasks together or even very occasionally doing some work for the client, where this is seen as appropriate for developing some contact and/or modelling an activity for the future benefit of the person.

Throughout this chapter I will attempt to examine the many functions and practical activities that may be employed with a view to assisting someone to cope, manage, fulfil ideas and wishes, but above all else to be in contact with valuable sources of helping. We are essentially looking at positive responses to people who are otherwise regarded as resistant or reluctant to have contact. The approach will be to firstly look at the initial engagement of a relationship and then to consider the elements for sustaining ongoing contact. Meanwhile we need to acknowledge a considerable degree of overlap between the practical strategies for initiating and those for sustaining the relationship.

DEFINITION OF 'ENGAGEMENT'

This is the process whereby a practitioner approaches a potential service user and/or carer as the first stage in establishing a trusting working relationship. It is an attempt to build something positive as a solid foundation for building an ongoing constructive partnership (Bleach, 1994).

For the practitioner a degree of successful engagement is necessary in order that the subsequent assessment, planning, implementing, monitoring and review functions of the professional process may be meaningful. Without this element of engagement these functions become rather biased towards the professional's view or even redundant if the client actively resists and avoids contact. For the client and the practitioner, the engagement of a positive relationship can become an intrinsic and beneficial element of the overall support, independent of any further practical interventions.

Kisthardt and Rapp (1989) assert that engagement should be viewed as a separate function in and of itself. This standpoint differentiates them from most of the professional approaches that acknowledge the need for a relationship but assume assessment to be the initial function of the professional process (Finlay, 1988).

Through the strengths model of case management, Kisthardt and Rapp (1989) suggest that engagement is about:

- educating or re-educating the client about the unique nature of support for their personal situation;
- helping the client to identify and realize their own wants and needs;
- the client and practitioner getting to know and to trust each other.

In this way, Kisthardt (1992) outlines a strengths model approach to engagement as taking the form of 'a series of unstructured, informal and conversational encounters that take place in the beginning of the helping process'.

Need for engagement

One aspect of the need has already been identified above, i.e. the necessity for engagement with a client to give meaning to all other aspects of the professional process, from assessment through to review of progress. Bleach (1994) suggests that 'Users may experience the relationship itself as therapeutic without there being any direct attempt at therapeutic activity beyond the establishing of the relationship'. Thus, there is an assumption that if therapeutic activity is indicated by the assessment and plan, engagement would be necessary before the construction of a plan but also as a modelling or demonstration technique to introduce the potential of therapeutic activities to the client and/or carer.

One of the principles of the strengths model of case management suggests that the relationship between the client and the case manager is the primary and essential factor in the helping process (Kisthardt, 1992; Onyett, 1992). The reasoning behind this principle focuses on the need for trust and cooperation in a partnership in order to achieve desired outcomes. It is widely understood that the client group build relationships only gradually and with reasonable initial feelings of uncertainty, doubt or even suspicion about the motives behind such relationships. Kisthardt and Rapp (1989) suggest that these responses should not necessarily be interpreted as symptoms of paranoia, 'But rather ... as a normal reaction to an uncertain and somewhat invasive interpersonal situation'.

Thus, we may see the process of engagement as a primary method of challenging mistrust and ambivalence about the potential of a positive relationship. It is necessary in order to effect the explanations needed to build confidence and trust in the support that may be offered.

Case study 5.1: Richard (46 years old)

Some details of Richard have already been discussed in Case Study 4.5. The essential points here are that his 22-year history of being diagnosed with manic depressive psychosis has brought him into repeated contact with psychiatric services, largely on an involuntary basis, generally offering him medical treatments that he doesn't want and does not see any need for. An additional difficulty is a recent council housing department ruling not to offer him a new tenancy until he proves his abilities in high supported accommodation; a decision which frustrates and angers him.

A simple referral was insufficient to involve Richard in a new type of service. He had long since lost his faith with services in general. A whole new approach of active engaging needed to be developed that would be responsive to his needs. The idea of informally listening to Richard's own account of his history, followed by an agreement to work together on his priority helped to inform him that support may be available that he could make some use of.

A subsequent use of team information leaflets helped to confirm the informal conversations about available support and Richard entered into a tentative negotiation of how he may use the services of a case manager in future.

IMPORTANCE OF THE FIRST MEETING

In traditional psychiatric services that uphold assessment to be the initial function of the process, the initial meeting frequently takes the more formal and structured approach. Such an approach may follow a stereotypical pattern with a controlled series of questions and answers. Some professionals may even refer to it formally as the 'initial interview'.

This approach is unlikely to hold much relevance for the majority of people in the long-term client group. They are likely to have had a good deal of prior contact with services and to have been through the formal initial assessment on many occasions before. Adopting such a hurried approach to information gathering is therefore unlikely to inform the client that you wish to offer a different type of service and may even alienate the client through perceived unresponsiveness to their needs.

Kanter (1989) reminds us that while some people may engage in services fairly rapidly over a matter of weeks or months, for some of the more vulnerable and disadvantaged clients the process may take several years before a stable and collaborative relationship is formed. For these reasons it is worth giving very careful consideration to the approach of the first meeting; it is rarely necessary to compile masses of information quickly and first impressions can create lasting impressions in the mind of the potential service user.

Above all else, we need to remember that it is the service providers that are establishing the need for a meeting in the first instance and rarely will it happen at the instigation of the client. As such, the client is quite within their rights to appear reluctant or suspicious – reactions which we should remember not to interpret as symptoms of illness (Kisthardt, 1992).

Preparation by practitioner

Kisthardt and Rapp (1989) remind us that the first meeting with a potential service user is a 'unique' occasion. You never have a second chance to make first impressions, so preparation for the event should be as thorough as possible. As we are generally considering people who have had some previous contact with services, it should be possible to gather a great deal of information in advance, thus reducing the need to put the client through the unnecessary task of answering a familiar string of factual questions. The source of referral and accessible records will provide much of the formal information to complete your own documentation, thus limiting or even eliminating the need for any formal paperwork to be used at the initial meeting.

The contacts with other people before meeting with the client should respect confidentiality, as a primary example of the respect you should accord to the client. Contact with other services will be governed by their respective policies and codes of practice on the release of information, but contact with carers, relatives or other associates of the client should be left until you have sought the client's permission. The exceptions would be if any of these carers happened to be the source of referral.

Significant information to be gathered in advance would include what Onyett (1992) refers to as 'issues of difference'. You should be aware, if possible, if the client may hold any prejudices against you, the worker, on the grounds of race, gender, age, sexuality, perceived class or physical appearance. Also, if there is the potential for communication difficulties through physical impairments or the need for an interpreter to overcome language barriers. Religious and cultural differences may also have an impact, e.g. visiting a Jewish client late Friday afternoon in winter, a time when the sabbath is due to commence.

It may be necessary to consider in advance where would be the best place for the meeting to happen. Is the client happy for a stranger to visit their home? What elements of risk could be involved for the worker, either from a client's reaction or the wider environment they live in? Is it an area considered unsafe due to other residents, dangerous dogs, faulty lifts and numerous flights of stairs? Will there be a need for more than one worker and if so, could it be two new people or a joint visit with the known referrer?

Part of the respect shown to the client may include finding out by what name they prefer being addressed by a stranger; first names are informal, but some people prefer the use of surnames until the formalities are completed. It is also more informal to introduce yourself by a first name, but this may not necessarily accord with the client's initial feelings about how they perceive the authority of people in official positions. It may help the whole process of introductions to find out the merit of an introductory letter or telephone call, where appropriate, to discuss a mutually convenient time and place for a face-to-face meeting.

The first meeting should be seen as an opportunity to share information, rather than simply for a practitioner to be gathering information in a one-sided fashion. In preparation, the practitioner may need to consider issues of boundaries and self-disclosure. Whilst the intention should be one of sharing, there is still a need to be mindful of the merits of presenting a friendly approach without necessarily slipping from a professional working relationship into that of friendship.

Bleach (1994) also reminds us to give some thought in advance to what levels of service may or may not be available to the client as we know them from the advance information we have been able to gather. This issue also reflects the inevitable power differential that will operate between a needy service user and the service provider. Such a degree of power and control can be potentially abused or misused in the particular approach of the worker. It is important to be aware of this differential and to plan ways of reducing its impact on a client in the first meeting.

Case study 5.2: John (60 years old)

Further details of John have been discussed in Case Study 1.1. In terms of the preparation for an initial meeting the first point was to consider the nature of the referral. John had been referred to case management services separately by his general practitioner (GP) and community psychiatric nurse (CPN). Both referrers had stressed John's reclusive and somewhat neglectful lifestyle and his frequent refusal to answer the door either to planned or spontaneous domiciliary visits. His long history of frequent relapses was largely attributed to this failure to maintain consistent contact with psychiatric services.

Preparation for the visit involved several important factors:

1. Discussions with referring agents elicited that John will not attend appointments at offices or clinics, but holds no fundamental objections to people visiting his home. It would be important to avoid clashing with the early afternoon daily visits to his local café.
2. The referral had been discussed with John by his CPN and he held no particular prejudices against any particular type of worker (by age, gender or race).
3. Researching John's extensive hospital medical notes gave detailed background information that eliminated the need for any formal questions in the first meeting.
4. The team policy was to allocate two workers for the early engagement period, partly to offer the client some choice in who may become primary keyworker but also to engage with a second worker for times of annual leave or sick leave cover.
5. It was apparent that John may not answer the door or be in favour of any lengthy meeting, so it was decided to send him an advance letter – informal greetings, introductions, time and date of proposed visit, a clause that he may cancel if the time was inconvenient without evoking any prejudicial feelings in the new workers. Reference was made to the referrers and that our meeting may only need to be a short friendly introduction.
6. Consideration of the potential plans that could be offered to John were left quite open, with an intended focus on encouraging him to discuss his own wants and wishes. A reference to using his local café was to be kept in mind as a way into informal discussion.

In the event, John had not bothered to open the letter, but he did allow the workers in on the basis that his CPN had discussed the referral with him. However, the letter was used informally to good effect as a method of introduction during the visit. The idea of using knowledge of the café also proved fortuitious, as John invited both workers to the café with him on their second visit.

The initial meeting

There is no simple formula for ensuring satisfactory engagement at a first meeting. Despite the attention to preparation it must always be borne in mind that a first meeting is an entirely unique situation. The client may not accept their need for help in quite the same way that the referrer has presented it. We should not make assumptions that a potential service user will be motivated to engage with us and perhaps more importantly, we should resist any temptation to attribute reluctance or resistance to symptoms of illness or personality traits. Bleach (1994) suggests that suspicion of services has been earned, as a result of previous experiences where services have failed to meet users' own perceptions of need. Kisthardt and Rapp (1989) suggest that such reluctance to engage is a quite normal human reaction to what is essentially a quite abnormal form of interpersonal relationship.

Onyett (1992) reminds us that even with advanced notice of the meeting we are still arriving as a stranger from nowhere and we need to help the client to place us in a more familiar context. For this reason it becomes important to make ourselves into a 'real person' by introducing our name rather than just our job title or details of the referral in the first exchange, though this other information will soon be necessary to help establish the context of the meeting. Introductions by name, in the first instance, help to personalize the process. The thinking behind this is that it is more difficult to instantly reject a name than it is to reject 'the social worker', for example.

The atmosphere of a first meeting should be carefully attended to, so that where possible the practitioner establishes a comfortable and positive ambience. Kisthardt and Rapp (1989) suggest that a non-threatening atmosphere is more easily established by focusing on topics of interest and concern to the client; to focus on the client's strengths, interests and abilities rather than the more usual inventory of problems. References to psychiatric history and symptomatology should be the prerogative of the client, not introduced immediately by the worker. You may feel it is appropriate to actively turn around the client's usual experience of such meetings, by rejecting the need to discuss the usual problems and actively drawing attention to positive interests.

A comfortable atmosphere may be engendered through an unstructured, informal and conversational approach by the practitioner. The tone of voice, rate of speech and active listening and attending to the client will help to promote the right atmosphere. Barriers may also be broken down by worker self-disclosure; this first meeting should be about the sharing of information and conversation, paying particular attention to the similarities as well as the differences of experience, (Morgan, 1993).

The practitioner should attempt to project a genuinely relaxed approach to engaging rather than the more pressured purpose of assessment. Bleach (1994) reminds us that formality should be something we occasionally opt in to, rather than occasionally opting out of. There is rarely a need to introduce paperwork in the initial meeting. The use of humour can have a powerful effect on promoting engagement but as discussed in Chapter 4, it needs to be very carefully judged so as not to offend or devalue the client.

The whole pace and direction of the meeting should ideally be dictated by the user themselves, though there are frequent occasions where they will expect to be led by the questioning of the worker, as a consequence of their previous experiences. The intention should be one of empowering the user to take an equal role in the interactions. Most clients will be unused to being offered power, control or choices about the priorities for the working relationship. In these circumstances the worker should be assertive in checking that the client understands what is being said or that they feel confident to participate effectively in the interactions. Morgan (1993) indicates that one aspect of empowering the user is to spend time determining similar agendas between the participants. The use of language can have a remarkable influence on the process. Use of professional jargon instantly skews the power relationship in favour of the worker; wherever possible you should endeavour to adopt the style and terminology of the client's language (Onyett, 1992).

If it is appropriate to discuss the nature of the services that can be offered, the primary quality from the worker should be that of honesty. Don't promise the earth, in the hope of promoting engagement by deception, as this will be gradually discovered through the subsequent succession of failed expectations.

Describe how the service works for the other users in similar circumstances, but be very clear about what is possible and what may not be. Your powers to access necessary resources may be limited or you may be bound by particular policies of the employing agency. Onyett (1992) suggests that, even with the limitations that restrict our abilities, we should 'get alongside the user' by demonstrating we are there for them rather than acting on behalf of other agencies.

Ultimately, we are trying to establish a role of providing a helping and supporting service for the potential user, but we should respect different perceptions and values or different behaviours demonstrated by the user. Have respect for their time and their privacy, particularly as you are likely to be the guest in their home or environment. Respect is demonstrated by arriving on time, resisting making rash promises, offering empathic understanding and acceptance of differences, by not attributing blame or trying unnecessarily to explain behaviour as symptoms and by not being quick to disagree with the client. Be aware and check out differences for yourself by considering if there are cultural, racial or spiritual reasons why the client may be seeing the world differently from you. There may be circumstances where you can honestly suggest to the client that you have much to learn from them and their circumstances. Potential service users can often recognize and appreciate respect and cooperation in place of their more usual perceptions of coercion.

One method of helping to initiate the relationship at a very early stage can be the offer of a practical task that may have fairly rapid and positive results. Practical tasks can have the benefit of demonstrating our intentions towards the client, even if they are not perceived as being a part of your usual role or even if they are the type of work that may be delegated to another person at a later stage. Witheridge (1989) suggests that an early aspect of engagement is likely to be assisting with a concrete task such as a financial or housing issue or even something as simple as cleaning in the home. Nothing breeds success quite like success and an increase in income or a reduction of debt can often be simple and quickly achieved with positive consequences for relationship building (Morgan, 1993). You are not buying cooperation if this is shown to be a small example of a broader plan for helping the client.

The question of boundaries is quite important in the first meeting, as it is for the longer term relationship. Self-disclosure has already been suggested as one method of 'being with' the client, but the guidelines around worker disclosures tend to be loose and open to personal interpretation. We need to be able to share something of ourselves in the same way as we expect clients to do to a much greater extent, but it is important to realize why you choose to divulge particular pieces of information. If a disclosure can be justified as helping a client's understanding then it remains valid but if its prime function has been the worker's relief, it is inappropriate. For example, if you use a real situation that has required the resolution of a difficulty in your own family – such as a child's schooling – it is appropriate as an illustration of problem solving, but not if it has served a primary function of offloading your own anxieties.

The ending of the initial meeting should be dictated by the actions of the client, where possible. The practitioner should attempt to make a positive and courteous ending note, with some agreement about the date, time and place of a further contact.

The client may end a meeting abruptly or only after a short period of time. These situations should be respected and accepted by the worker and seen as an active expression of power and choice by the service user. There may be circumstances where the user's general mistrust of service intentions leads them to test out the worker who is making somewhat different approaches and promises; this should not be automatically seen as rejection by the worker.

All of the above discussion assumes that the potential service user is not assessed to be at risk in any way, to themselves, the worker or others. Part of the preparation may have involved a decision to make the first contact with somebody who is already well known to the client – the referrer, a relative or friend perhaps. The worker always has a duty of care to assess risk and may on some occasions need to take more urgent action if somebody is found to be at some significant risk at the first meeting, e.g. actively suicidal or threatening intent. Indeed, it could be useful quite early in the relationship to be very clear that your role is to work with the client's wishes but that you have a duty to override these wishes if you can demonstrate a potential or actual serious risk to the client or others.

Case study 5.3: Marianne (53 years old)

This lady had experienced a 25-year history of being diagnosed with schizophrenia. She also suffered several physical complaints, many attributed to excessive smoking and obesity, with a sedentary lifestyle. Marianne had been referred to case management services by her social worker, with the request for intensive support for a lady who had become very chaotic and neglectful of herself and her flat.

It had been decided, after contact with the referrer, that two case managers would make the initial contact with Marianne at her home. This plan had been discussed by the referrer with Marianne and had received her agreement.

The initial contact took the form of a semi-naked Marianne greeting the two visitors through an open letterbox. Initial introductions were kept to first names and brief reference to the social worker by first name only. Care was taken to protect Marianne's privacy and feelings, by not openly discussing outside the flat that this visit was the psychiatric services calling to see her.

After adjusting her clothing, Marianne did invite the case managers into the flat with immediate apologies about the condition of it, that she hadn't found time to tidy up before the meeting. Every surface, item of furniture and floor was covered or strewn with items of clothing, shopping and food, including cat food. Six chicken carcasses were counted on the kitchen and living room floors alone. You had to watch your step!

Much of the discussion that ensued took place with the case managers precariously standing in the living room and Marianne smoking on her bed in an adjoining room, surrounded by half-eaten snacks and mountains of cigarette ends. The challenge was to engage Marianne without resorting to a rapid assessment based solely on the condition of the flat.

With some value judgements suspended, the discussion focused positively on Marianne's interests in shopping and cooking and her cat. The case managers were able to demonstrate a practical role for helping by cleaning away some of the accumulated food on the floors.

Failure and follow-up

The initial approach to establishing contact with a potential service user may frequently result in a very short and apparently unproductive meeting or a forthright refusal to meet or simply no response at all. It is important to avoid instantly negative conclusions, but to once again be aware that reluctance or resistance to your well-intentioned approaches arises from a much greater experience of failed expectations, inappropriate service responses and steadily built mistrust and scepticism. These are not circumstances that can be rapidly turned around.

Onyett (1992) suggests not only that we learn to respect a user's initial negative reactions towards us, but also that we ultimately need to respect the right to refuse offers of help and support. Unless there is a clearly defined assessment of risk to themselves or others, the user can deny the need for any external help. Bleach (1994) suggests that in these circumstances case management services have frequently developed a compromise between respecting these wishes and developing more creative approaches to engage by different methods or at least making an effort to ensure some form of contact for users who may change their minds subsequently. This creativity and compromise enables workers to sustain motivation at times of rejection. Maintaining initial contacts with carers, neighbours or friends of the user, within bounds of confidentiality, may enable indirect contact and support to be sustained.

Kisthardt and Rapp (1989) have identified that some users will engage rapidly with services, while others take much longer. For some users it may well be a method of 'testing out' the intentions or promises of the worker. Case management services attempt to demonstrate how they are different from other services but this difference may need to be tested in some way in order for some users to develop confidence in it.

It is important that the worker does not overanalyse the possible reasons for failure, as this all too often results in the search for causes in the client or the attribution to personality factors, which can ultimately be destructive to further attempts to engage the user. We generally find it more difficult to acknowledge the causes or problems in ourselves and our own working practice (Morgan, 1993).

The use of individual supervision and team discussions can promote creativity in establishing new methods of engagement. Ultimately, we acknowledge and communicate that the user is engaging with the team rather than the individual worker; in some situations this may help to alleviate some of the user's concerns about engaging with a particular individual.

Onyett (1992) suggests that we may need to 'try another tack', by passing the job of engagement on to another worker without feeling a loss of face. Alternatively, it may be a case of offering an appointment to meet at a different venue if the user has felt uncertain or ambivalent about the original plans.

Practical interventions may take a number of forms, but it may ultimately depend on persistence of the worker. Some evidence suggests that service users recognize and respond to the caring notion underpinning perseverance and that this can be an important element of establishing a relationship (Ford *et al.*, 1993). Onyett (1992) suggests that we may wish to persist even at times when the client has refused contact, but that it may be appropriate to simply leave a name and a contact number for when the person has a change of mind about the possibilities of contact. It becomes necessary for the practitioner to work more at an intuitive level, because a number of decisions may be necessary about direct or indirect contact, the wider assessment of risks and the rights of the individual to take risks and make mistakes as a part of their own learning process.

The question of using indirect contacts raises a number of practical options for services. Letters, phone calls or dropping a note through the door when passing, provided they are not construed as harassment, can be potential methods of demonstrating that we do care for the client (Kisthardt and Rapp, 1989) and fulfil our intentions of offering longer term support, not just a brief contact for assessment (Morgan, 1993). We may maintain our indirect contact by linking with known and trusted others who continue to have direct contact with the client or we may set up a joint visit with another known and trusted person.

Continued visits to the client's home may help us to build some knowledge of useful details, even if direct contact is not achieved with much success. Again, the issue of harassment needs to be carefully assessed, but we may develop knowledge of the telltale signs of someone in residence or out, e.g. John (in Case Study 5.2) uses a specific configuration of internal door opening and closing which indicates if he is home or not, which can be seen from his letterbox. At time when John does not answer the door it is possible to determine whether he is home or not. Other people may have their own methods, whether by positioning of curtains or arrangement of personal items viewed in a passageway through a letterbox. If we have any cause to be concerned about a person's well-being but receive no answer to our visits, a very discreetly placed wedge of card or paper in between door and frame may at least indicate if the door has been opened between visits.

One practical method that needs to be very carefully considered before being attempted is the use of deception or hijack. Deception in the strictest sense is very dangerous, but we may try to see someone 'accidentally' at a place known to be used by the client, e.g. café or shopping area. Whilst this may succeed in establishing contact and can have a long-term benefit in the process of engagement, it can equally be very damaging if a client subsequently feels they have been tricked or deceived into contact.

Case study 5.4: Reginald (54 years old)

This gentleman was known to be living an agoraphobic existence at home with his elderly disabled mother. The referral to case management by his GP stressed a psychotic diagnosis, but with a concern that he had not been outside his flat for over 20 years and presented extreme vulnerability in view of his mother's precarious health.

Initial contact, following a letter, was met by a brief but abusive rejection of services through a closed door. The assessment of vulnerability and inadequate ability to support his ageing mother led to a decision to persist with attempts to establish contact. Reginald persisted in his refusal to open the front door, but his frequent abusive rejections of the advances to him were interspersed with comments that suggested he was acknowledging the contact, e.g. 'Don't call back for another two weeks!'.

These brief encounters through a closed door continued for 18 months, in the knowledge that indirect contact could also be maintained through discussions with the district nursing service who were gaining entry daily to treat Reginald's mother.

Individual supervision and team discussions helped to sustain this plan in the face of continual rejection and occasional abuse. Ultimately, Reginald's mother had to be hospitalized and subsequently died but for him the precedent of indirect contact had an unquantifiable effect and he was subsequently able to tolerate direct contact from another service responding to his grief and isolation.

SUSTAINING LONG-TERM RELATIONSHIPS

Many of the factors discussed in relation to the establishing of the initial engagement are equally as valid for the sustaining and development of that relationship. Many writers have suggested that a fully engaged relationship with a client experiencing long-term mental health problems can take many years to establish. This is particularly the case with people who, for very good reasons, are resistant or reluctant to engage with services that have generally failed to satisfy needs as they perceive them personally. These people will take a great deal of winning over, by a patient worker supporting them through relapses of personal difficulties and essentially proving themselves as a trusted contact.

Such a prospect can have a draining effect on a worker who, though committed to the provision of a high quality and responsive service, still needs to perpetually prove themselves. Morale and motivation can be easily sapped. Bleach (1994) points out a number of factors that may aid the worker in sustaining meaningful working relationships, but also support their own morale and motivation: realism, a long-term perspective, positive understanding and user-centred flexibility. Other factors will be discussed subsequently, including some of the issues around the degree and the quality of engagement.

Realism

Realistic expectations and the setting of small, achievable goals help the user and worker alike to acknowledge successes and offset the frustration of failure when we set higher or more global aims. A role for the practitioner is one of negotiating a path between under- and overexpectations on behalf of self, user, carers and other services. Realism aids the process of engagement by demonstrating serious consideration of the user's potentials and by helping the practitioner to be clear and honest about their own resources and potentials.

Long-term perspective

This involves the practitioner helping the user to see beyond the present crisis to hold onto the more stable and sustainable long-term goals. Such a perspective allows for the occasional setbacks to be seen in context as only a small part of a longer term constructive process for change. It may also enable the practitioner to adopt a more relaxed attitude towards the occasional tensions between the professional view of the need for support and the user view of resisting the advances of unnecessary service interventions.

Positive empathic understanding

The skill of empathy has been addressed in Chapter 4. It essentially entails working through the service user's own terms, being with them, empowering them to participate equally in the whole process of support. Understanding situations the way the user experiences them can also help the practitioner to understand the reasons for what may be seen as unpredictable, chaotic and resistant behaviours. The development of positive empathic understanding can be learned by an individual practitioner, but it is also clearly supported by a positive 'team culture' of regard for service users.

User-centred flexibility

This factor draws our attention to a philosophical change from the service-centred notion of 'What have we got available and how will the client be able to make use of it?' to a much more individualized notion of 'What does the client want and need and how can we access the resources to meet these ideas?'. The 'take it or leave it' view of service provision has frequently failed the service user with long-term complex needs. Furthermore, such a limited approach does little to persuade a person of the desirability of a service.

Flexibility allows the provision of service more on user terms and it also enables the practitioner to generate their own motivations through extending and crossing boundaries of professional practice in order to meet the needs expressed. However, the notion of realism also needs to be applied here to the limits of flexibility: individual practitioners need to be aware of their own limitations as well as those imposed by policies and culture of the employing agency.

Human and technical skills

A wide range of learned skills may be employed for sustaining the development of a working relationship, but in a number of studies service users have drawn attention to the more human and personalized approaches offered by their individual case manager (Kisthardt, 1992; Cooke et al., 1994). The characteristics commonly referred to in a helper were: warm, accepting, understanding, involved, natural, genuine, competent, self-disclosing.

Consistency of personnel

From a user's perspective the greater the continuity of their service personnel the more satisfactory is the process of engaging. A frequently expressed criticism of psychiatric services is the rapid turnover of staff: 'Just when you are getting to know your worker they leave!'. This factor is essential when we consider the earlier comment regarding the potential timescale of engagement stretching into years.

It is difficult to commit your trust to someone who is not likely to be with you for long or to a rapid succession of different people. The retention of staff is a separate issue that is affected by employers' attitudes and policies. One approach adopted by many teams is that of engaging a potential service user with the team, through the initial contacts of one team member. The use of team and client shared outings, a groupwork programme or a clients' Christmas party can be of benefit for introducing clients to other workers in the service. However, the quality of engagement is still likely to differ between the worker seen on a weekly basis and other team members seen less often and possibly at a more superficial level.

Empowerment and dependency

Many service users will respond to a service that actively promotes their independence in making choices and decisions about their own futures. This aspect will be discussed in more detail in Chapter 6. However, at times of crisis or acute distress, when a condition is taking a turn for the worse and decisions seem to be too much of a burden, it can be useful to know that you can rely on a case manager or keyworker to offer the kind of help and support that still respects your longer term independence.

Collusion

In general, the practice of colluding with a client's delusional beliefs should not be encouraged, as the potential for reinforcing symptoms could result in perpetuating the individual's experience of distress.

However, all rules can be challenged by exceptional circumstances and there are certainly occasions where to challenge a client's delusional beliefs will result in an instant loss of any engaged relationship. For this reason, it is important to carefully evaluate the individual circumstances and closely monitor the effects of any implied collusion if this tack is taken in order to promote engagement. This is particularly significant where the loss of contact may be viewed as a potential for risk to the client or others. However, the approach adopted should favour a playing down of the challenge to beliefs rather than an active embracing of the delusional ideas by the worker.

Involvement in reviews

The process of monitoring and review can appear quite alien to clients and intrinsic to the professionalization of approaches. For many the use of paperwork and the formality of meetings can be a burden they would rather leave to workers. However, many users can be empowered to cooperate in the review of progress and to set their own agendas for future change. The onus should be on the worker adopting creative methods to make the whole review process less formal and more user-friendly.

DEGREE OF ENGAGEMENT

This may reflect the complexity of user needs and the complexity of potential service responses, as well as the interactions of motivations to engage between users and practitioners (Bleach, 1994).

Where the requirements for service input are clear and uncontroversial there is a potential need for a coordination role but less intensive direct contact and need for engagement. Where the requirement is one of building complex plans around the service user's wishes and needs, where it is a case of challenging suspicion and resistance, then the need for engagement becomes more crucial for developing long-term interventions for support.

As we have already seen, a creative approach will recognize the respective value of engaging with the user, carers and other services. It is quite possible that the contact can be maintained more intensively with informal carers, whilst keeping contact and possible frustration to a minimum with the client.

Case study 5.5: Peter (36 years old)

Peter experiences psychiatric services only as a result of the legal process, following arrests for petty criminal offences and subsequent court assessment eliciting mental health difficulties at the time of the offences.

His view is clear and consistent, that services are only intent on giving him medication and no further support or understanding of his wants and needs.

Peter's suspicion of others, whether it be his family, neighbours or case manager, extends to rarely opening the door to visitors. Much of this suspicion has to be seen in the context of very real racial harassment from other people on his inner-city council estate.

Peter's family have their own agreement to hold a spare key to his flat, to offer regular support even in the face of his occasional abusive responses. The family are in regular contact with the case manager, acting as a channel for the mail around Peter's housing and financial affairs. In this way the case manager has been enabled to offer a level of service to Peter with only minimal direct contact. Peter is aware of these circumstances and the continuing situation whereby he has not merely been persuaded to use medication as a solution to his living conditions. As a result, the infrequent direct contacts between Peter and his case manager have assumed a lesser degree of suspicion.

QUALITY OF THE RELATIONSHIP

As with the degree of engagement, the quality of the interpersonal contacts can vary substantially but they need to be analysed for their deeper potential, not just superficially valued or devalued for any reason. There is no baseline of interpersonal communication that reflects a qualitative value on the relationship. Some people take an instant positive view of a worker showing interest in them, with volumes of information and feelings being disclosed. Others act much more cautiously on their learned suspicion and mistrust of service approaches; guarded in communication, withholding of the more meaningful information, determining only specific areas of interest that they will engage in or allow discussion or support in.

The latter position is to be respected and where possible worked with creatively to gain the inherent quality. By adjusting our own expectations we may see that with many people in the client group maintenance of contact is all that is needed. Deeper meaningful communication may be a bonus in some situations, but a continuing contact can have a recognized qualitative element to supporting a person and their wishes.

Case study 5.6: Mary (58 years old)

Mary lives alone since the death of her husband four years ago. Her main experience of psychiatric services is a 20-year hospital admission in one of the old institutions.

Her only desire is to keep living in her flat (despite the view of others that she experiences persistent symptoms of thought disorder and is very neglectful of herself and her environment).

The case management services have been proactive in refurbishing Mary's flat for continued habitation in recent years, following a severe flood from upstairs and years of neglect of decor and furnishings.

Mary has been continuously reluctant to permit access to her flat, partly through guarding her own privacy and partly from fear of people wishing to return her to hospital. She is aware of the need to permit brief daily access to district nurses to monitor her medication. However, Mary can be verbally abusive to visitors and ends visits on the doorstep abruptly after only a few seconds.

Through three years of occasional verbal abuse (with occasional spontaneous apologies) from Mary the case manager has managed to negotiate regular contact and a liaison role between Mary and other services (medical, meals-on-wheels and financial). Frequent reassurances that all is being done to help Mary to enjoy living at home have aided the continuation of these contacts. Despite the very short duration of contact, the quality lies in the development of support that is flexible to Mary's needs and thus maintains her at home.

ISSUES OF 'DIFFERENCE'

There are many issues that may throw up the differences between a service user and a worker. The cultural, racial and gender differences will be discussed in Chapter 7, but we also need to attend here to the occasions when differences are likely to occur over the issue of service need. The two most clear examples of difference occur over the formal detention of a client and the administration of injectable medications.

Roles have been clearly defined for social workers and nurses in the above examples, but when we are considering the engagement of a long-term relationship, definitions drawn up solely along the lines of professional responsibility are not always going to encourage the potentially reluctant service user.

As in all aspects of the work in helping people with complex long-term needs, the individual situation needs to be assessed independently. There are occasions when the keyworker or case manager, being seen as closely associated with procedures to detain under the Mental Health Act, will be viewed with hostility and it may be politic to take a coordinating role at an 'invisible distance'. However, it may also be worth considering a directly supportive role, being seen as the person who reminded you about the need to take the cigarettes and the change of clothing with you; being the supportive person in the community who was prepared to follow you with this support into the hospital. Some people have subsequently valued such support.

A similar level of individual consideration needs to be given to the potentially emotive issue of depot injections. Some users may not see the giving of their injection as being in any way detrimental to their wider relationship with a service worker. However, the client group is characterized by issues of resistance over depot injections. In these situations it may be very damaging to a wider supportive relationship to be seen as the person giving the unwanted or painful injection. Options for community psychiatric nurses may include engaging the services of other nurses to give injections to their clients, e.g. depot clinics, GP practices, team colleagues. Similarly, you may be called upon to give the injections to clients of other team colleagues, in some form of reciprocal arrangement.

ASSERTIVE OUTREACH

This method of working is frequently assumed by community services to be a flexible and proactive way of ensuring that people do not 'fall through the cracks' and fail to receive a service simply because they are too disturbed, too resistant or too unreachable. It usually describes a policy of taking positive action to reach people rather than waiting for them to come and seek services (Bleach, 1994).

Kisthardt and Rapp (1989) suggest that engagement is fostered by the principle of assertive outreach. They see it as a collaborative response to service delivery, taking services to where the client feels most comfortable to make use of them. The opposite approach has been the much used and least successful notion of 'take it or leave it'. Many people who feel inclined to 'leave it' are often seen to be at high risk of returning to hospital on a regular basis – the revolving door clients.

Service providers are generally more motivated towards the potential benefits of their services than are many of the people in the client group so services need to follow clients, rather than blandly expecting them to attend appointments at offices, clinics and centres. Kisthardt (1992) suggests that service users can be seen to be voting with their feet by staying away from many of the structured programmes that are developed for them. Hagan (1990) lists the reasons for non-attendance as disaffection, poor memory, difficulties with structuring time, communication difficulties, lack of information, stigma, inaccessibility, unwelcoming and culturally insensitive services.

Despite the apparent advantages assertive outreach is still a controversial policy for service delivery. A key issue appears to be the dilemma of finding a balance between a user's right to refuse contact and the practitioner's responsibility of providing a service to a person who may be at risk of neglect, self-injury or of harming others (Bleach, 1994). Users have a right to make their own decisions, their own choices, to take some degree of risk and make mistakes just like anyone else.

The answer seems to lie in a distinction between the active engaging process involved in 'assertive' outreach, as opposed to more coercive and enforcing implications of 'aggressive' outreach. If we are positively seeking to present acceptable and desirable services responsive to client need, the dilemma naturally diminishes. Kisthardt and Rapp (1989) suggest that by allowing clients to determine where service delivery can take place we send a clear message that they have a collaborative and empowering role to play in directing the helping process. A flexible approach to assertive outreach even enables some users to make the initial contacts in service settings rather than their own environments, if this feels safer and more acceptable (Kisthardt, 1992).

Bleach (1994) suggests that users must retain the right to say no, but that practitioners need to be flexible in gauging how quickly, literally and absolutely to respond to each refusal. We always need to bear in mind the assessments of risk. External advocacy services may have a role to play in supporting users' rights to say no.

SUMMARY

The focus of the supportive relationship is on establishing and maintaining contact between service providers and potential service users. We are primarily concerned with engaging clients who for many different reasons have not previously experienced services as positively responding to their needs. Reluctance or resistance on behalf of a client should not be immediately perceived as a symptom; it is a quite normal reaction to a rather abnormal social interaction (Kisthardt, 1992).

We need to view the engagement process as an entirely separate function of our work. The very first meeting is a unique event and this can be acknowledged by focusing our attention onto the person's strengths, abilities, interests and their expressed priorities (Kisthardt and Rapp, 1989). We should be prepared to engage with people by working alongside them on very practical tasks (Witheridge, 1989), not necessarily being seen as the agent of the purely medical psychological approaches to assessing potential problems.

Degrees of engagement and the quality of the developing relationship may be promoted through the functions of assertive outreach. This is a method of delivery that takes the service out to the client, following them into their community, rather than expecting them to attend the services. However, the policy of assertive outreach poses a controversial dilemma: whilst it potentially empowers the involvement of service users, it can also raise serious questions about the tension between assessing levels of risk and accepting a user's right to refuse contact (Bleach, 1994).

REFERENCES

Bleach, A. (1994) *'Engagement' Draft Training Module*, Sainsbury Centre for Mental Health, London.

Cooke, A., Repper, J., Ford, R. *et al.* (1994) *Assorted Interviews during the RDP/DoH Research*, Research and Development for Psychiatry, London.

Finlay, L. (1988) *Occupational Therapy Practice in Psychiatry*, Croom Helm, London.

Ford, R., Repper, J., Cooke, A. *et al.* (1993) *Implementing Case Management*, Research and Development for Psychiatry, London.

Hagan, T. (1990) Accessible and acceptable services in *Effective Community Mental Health Services,* (ed. P. Huxley), Avebury/Gower, Aldershot.

Kanter, J. (1989) Clinical case management: definition, principles, components. *Hospital and Community Psychiatry,* **40**(4), 361–8.

Kisthardt, W.E. (1992) A strengths model of case management: the principles and functions of a helping partnership with persons with persistent mental illness, in *A Strengths Perspective for Social Work Practice,* (ed. D. Saleeby), Longman, New York, pp. 59–83.

Kisthardt, W.E. and Rapp, C.A. (1989) *Bridging the Gap Between Principles and Practice: Implementing a Strengths Perspective in Case Management*, University of Kansas, Lawrence.

Morgan, S. (1993) *Community Mental Health: Practical Approaches to Long-Term Problems,* Chapman & Hall, London.

Onyett, S. (1992) *Case Management in Mental Health*, Chapman & Hall, London.

Pilling, S. (1991) *Rehabilitation and Community Care*, Routledge, London.

Witheridge, T.F. (1989) The assertive community treatment worker: an emerging role and its implications for professional training. *Hospital and Community Psychiatry,* **40**(6), 620–4.

FURTHER READING

Bleach, A. and Ryan, P. (1995) *Community Support for Mental Health. A Handbook for the Care Programme Approach and Care Management.* Sainsbury Centre for Mental Health and Pavilion Publishing, Brighton.

Grunebaum, H. and Friedman, H. (1988) Building collaborative relationships with families of the mentally ill. *Hospital and Community Psychiatry,* **39**(11), 1183–7.

Perkins, R. and Dilks, S. (1992) Worlds apart: working with severely socially disabled people. *Journal of Mental Health,* **1**, 3–17.

Repper, J., Ford, R. and Cook, A. (1994) How can nurses build trusting relationships with people who have severe and long-term mental health problems? Experiences of case managers and their clients. *Journal of Advanced Nursing,* **19**, 1096–104.

6 | User empowering relationships

The concepts of advocacy and user empowerment have progressively developed over the last decade in the UK. From what might initially have been accepted as interesting ideas in the theoretical sense, they have now developed into what is acknowledged to be a vital aspect of the complex partnerships that drive service organization and change. Service users, whether at the individual or collective level, have had to struggle and fight to have their views on service provision heard, let alone accepted and acted upon. Arguably, the 1980s focus on consumerism and market forces offered an unexpected external political impetus, which has reinforced the importance of the service users' views.

Much of the discussion and publication of ideas has so far concentrated on the collective responsibilities at the 'user movement' and 'service organization' levels. The early accounts were generated by the work of users themselves (Chamberlain, 1988; Beeforth *et al.*, 1990) but more recently service providers have also sought to recognize such developments in print (MIND, 1992a; Morgan, 1993). References to empowering the individual have tended to be less frequent and usually in the context of illustrating the broader concepts.

In this chapter, I will attempt to translate many of the service level theories into ideas, values and practices that are meaningful to the individual user-provider working relationship.

In one sense, it is easier to talk of initiatives at the service organization level, because it can feel safer to contemplate the potential for change from a theoretical perspective couched in the terms of policy directives, projecting the allure of seductive jargon, protected by the cover of collective responsibility. Real change and empowerment in practice must ultimately arise from individual responsibility, at the point where a service impinges directly on the experience of the individual user.

By way of illustration, I would suggest that the collective responsibility focuses on issues such as user representation on decision-making panels or service planning groups, on recruitment panels, on the training and development of professional groups, on evaluation of services and also on the drawing up and publicizing of guidelines for practitioners. The individual worker responsibility should implement these guidelines in practice, by helping each service user to feel valued, unique, informed and with the power to exercise choices and decisions regarding all aspects of their own daily lives.

The reasons why the views of mental health service users should be taken seriously have been outlined by Rogers *et al.* (1993):

1. Attention to the views of users of psychiatric services has not kept pace with that of other groups of users of healthcare services.
2. People experiencing long-term severe mental health problems will probably have far more extensive contact with health services.
3. The labelling and stigma that accompany a psychiatric diagnosis such as schizophrenia will have a much greater negative impact on the life of the individual.

Some of the terminology used to refer to the organization of services should probably be clarified at this point, for fear of the potential misuse and confusion of terms.

- 'Service-centred' organization refers to a predominantly appointment-based system, where the individual user would be expected to attend a clinic, centre or office to meet with a service provider. Except in exceptional circumstances, decisions are made for the purpose of service efficiency, the user is expected to be flexible to service organization needs and any criticism of the organization is likely to be met with defensive statements about the volume of workload necessitating such an arrangement.
- 'Client-centred' organization refers more to the practices and decisions of the worker attempting to reflect the real or perceived needs of the individual user. The organization will aim for a much greater outreach perspective and flexibility of its own arrangements.
- 'User-led' organization is not the same as the 'client centred' approach. This is where the choices, decisions and possibly provision of the service are entirely in the control of users. It should logically meet, rather than reflect, real needs and changing needs. Service perceptions of need should not play any influencing role. An example of user-led services would be 'consciousness-raising' meetings, excluding all non-users of services (professionals and carers).

What I will primarily be concerned with in this chapter is the client-centred organizational approach to the individual service user. Beeforth *et al.* (1994), in conducting their own independent user evaluation of the Sainsbury Centre for Mental Health case management initiative, have highlighted the value of a meaningful individual relationship as the central notion of a client-centred approach to health and social care. It is seen to reflect the important ideas of 'partnership in care' and the user's desire to be listened to. These ideas correlate quite closely to views expressed in Chapter 5 about how service users recognize and appreciate cooperation rather than coercion. Also how service providers are valued if they are seen to be genuinely working alongside the individual user, rather than as an agent of others or the employing authority.

Before going on to examine the whole concept of 'power', I would like you to briefly consider the following two fictitious case scenarios in the light of cooperation', 'coercion' and a sense of 'empowerment'.

Situation one

Ms X attends an outpatient clinic for appointment with Dr Y, presenting with feelings of tiredness and distressing thoughts. Dr Y states that he will need to ask the questions that will help him to determine a diagnosis and the prescription of treatment. Tablets are prescribed and Ms X is asked to come back in one month to review progress.

At the follow-up appointment Ms X reports that the distressing thoughts persist, her sleep pattern is settling but is still of intermittent quality, but she now experiences additional senses of nausea and irritability of mood. She expresses a wish to stop the tablets. Dr Y suggests that there are signs the medication is doing some good, but maybe with some slight side-effects. He decides to prescribe tablets to tackle the side-effects and also an additional medication to speed the control of the disturbing thoughts.

Ms X subsequently feels persistently drowsy and lethargic, the troublesome thoughts decrease but she has a sense of powerlessness to control her life and quite alone with her feelings.

Situation two

Ms R attends an outpatient clinic for appointment with Dr S, presenting with feelings of tiredness and distressing thoughts. Dr S explains that such a combination is relatively common, but often with very individual causes depending on personal circumstances and exposure to stresses. It will be important for the two of them to talk, to help decide the possible causes and to look together at the choices of treatment that may be available.

Dr S suggests that medication may provide short-term relief of the distress and some undisturbed sleep, but that it could also present side-effects A, B or C, which should be reported back immediately, so they can discuss whether Ms R wishes to continue with these particular tablets. Dr S also discusses the option of seeing a counsellor to investigate the causes of stress further and the possibility of longer term employment retraining as an option that could benefit Ms R's particular situation. Ms R is asked to return in one month to review the medication and discuss her decisions about the other choices.

At the follow-up appointment Ms R decides to stop the medication as her sleep pattern is beginning to settle. She feels the option of counselling could be more beneficial for looking into her experiences of distress, but wishes to hold open the decision about future skills retraining until after the counselling. Dr S makes the referral to the counsellor, stops the medication and offers another appointment to come to see him. Ms R continues to experience distressing thoughts, but also feels she has some options and good advice to pursue.

POWER

In relation to the individual user of mental health services, the concept of power relates to control over the exercising of choice and the ability to make decisions regarding personal daily living needs. This ranges from the basic day-to-day needs essential for life (e.g. eating, drinking and sleeping) to the complex decisions regarding personal status through accommodation, activity and social relationship.

Wills (1982) reminds us that people experiencing mental health problems generally only consult services at times of illness, disability or acute difficulties. At this point there is already an implicit power differential established between the needy service user and the professional service provider. A person experiencing mental distress, with potentially disturbing symptoms, loss of role and status, difficulty with interpersonal relationships and possible decreased financial security, will tend to see very few areas of their life where they can exercise control. Read and Wallcraft (1992) also highlight the feelings of powerlessness and loss of control experienced by a person at the point where they feel a need to seek out help. However, far from supporting the regaining of control, they suggest that practitioners frequently reinforce the problem by disempowering the service user even further. This point is illustrated in 'Situation One' above, resulting in the service provider adopting a somewhat paternalistic control over treatment decisions and choices available to the person presenting in distress.

Empowerment and enablement

Stewart (1994) links these two concepts to show how the principle of power sharing can be effected in practice. She points to empowerment being about control and choice, participation and consultation, but the ability of the individual user to make full use of empowerment is through the practical functions of 'enablement'.

> Enablement is about helping the individual to achieve what is important to that person, and not necessarily about seeking normality or conformity. It is about helping people to respond to their circumstances; to assert their individuality and establish their goals. It is about establishing cooperative relationships. It is about removing barriers and creating opportunities which will help individuals to explore new areas, develop skills and gain mastery over their environment in keeping with their own aspirations.
>
> *(Stewart, 1994, p. 248)*

The emphasis on personal choice and achieving aspirations or desired goals will be developed further in this chapter when we consider the practical implementation of the strengths model of case management. Certainly the central theme of empowering the individual should focus on how the service provider is able to adapt to the expressed wishes of the individual user, rather than the more traditional disempowering nature of services that expect the individual to fit in where they are placed, to achieve the service-orientated statement of goals.

However, this more empowering direction, whereby the individual practitioner asks for and acts on the stated priorities of the service user, requires a major shift in the attitudes of the professional. It requires less emphasis on the implicit role and functions of the 'expert' and certainly a substantial modification of the traditional expert-sick role relationship. Hutchinson *et al.* (1990) remind us that such a switch to more user-empowering relationships need not threaten professional skills. More importantly, it asks the practitioner to prioritize different professional skills or to use their skills in a different way: working with people, listening and attending (Chapter 4), establishing jointly agreed care plans and developing individualized networks of support.

Information sharing

The mechanism on which power is based is 'information'. The implicit power differential between a service user and a practitioner hinges on the assumption that training and qualifications give the latter information not possessed by the service user, who brings the illness and distress ingredients to the working relationship. Wills (1982) suggests that the sharing of information is vital to the development of a positive relationship. The withholding of information sets up expectations of uncertainty and an increased sense of anxiety and distress. Hutchinson *et al.* (1990) state we cannot give an individual power in a literal sense, but if we acknowledge that information represents power we can give over the information.

The user of services wishing to regain some control over their personal circumstances should be encouraged to exercise choices and make decisions. This ability will be determined by the levels of information, awareness and education that are promoted by the service practitioner. The user's need for information will focus on a number of areas, including:

- the meaning of diagnostic labels;
- the identification of causal factors and early warning signs;
- the use of medication, potential side-effects and prognosis;
- the roles of different professionals;
- the range of potential services available;
- the service policies on such things as confidentiality and access to information;
- the service user's rights to and within services, including access to complaints procedures and service advocacy.

Information and education should not be restricted simply to medical aspects of care. Causal factors for episodes of distress present an area of potential conflict, whereby the practitioner often focuses on the medical health possibilities and the individual user will more frequently emphasize the social and environmental influences. Housing conditions, financial difficulties, occupational and recreational opportunities and the impact of interpersonal relationships may all have an influence on the potential for distress. All areas should be considered in the process of information sharing and education. Furthermore, it is important for the sharing of power to acknowledge the information and teaching roles and potentials of the individual service user, particularly in relation to their own experience of distress and use of services. Awareness and information sharing should be acknowledged as a two-way process within the working relationship.

Language

Information is power, but for it to be meaningful it needs to be freely accessible, complete and presented in an understandable format. Our own use of language, particularly jargon, needs to be addressed when we are presenting information to the service user for them to make informed choices. Beeforth *et al.* (1990) suggest that the use of professional jargon is a method of disguising information, allowing it to be shared only with a selected group of people who can understand the specialized language.

The consequence of this situation for an individual is an inevitable sense of powerlessness, feeling excluded and maybe even intimidated. It may also leave the person feeling that their situation is entirely their own fault, reinforced by a failure to understand the language being used. Take a moment now to remember how you personally felt the last time you were in a group of people and didn't understand the meaning of a particular word or phrase; we do not all have the confidence to ask for a meaning if we perceive ourselves to be the only one in ignorance.

Hutchinson *et al.* (1990) suggest that professional jargon is wholly unnecessary; that everything can be said in quite simple and under-standable terms. The onus should not be placed on the individual user to learn the language, but on the practitioner to return to the language of the real world, the world they generally inhabit when outside the profes-sional role!

Case study 6.1: Patrick (54 years old)

Diagnosed with schizophrenia and suffering frequent epileptic fits, Patrick has had contact with local psychiatric services for approx-imately 30 years. Due to various behavioural disturbances including verbal aggression towards staff, Patrick has been banned from attending some services and is bound by behavioural contracts at the one day centre he wishes to continue contact with. Patrick shares a flat with his 90-year-old mother, who experiences many physical disabilities and spells of depression.

Choices and decisions
Patrick acknowledges his own mood changes, but sees his behaviour towards representatives of services as justified because the years of contact have generally left him feeling frustrated because of his inability to return to work. He now maintains some control over the frequency of contact with the day centre (though less control over his activity while there), and total control over the personnel who may visit his home. He maintains a strong desire to care for his mother and for the two of them to refuse the offer of some 'elderly services' to the home. Patrick holds the office telephone number of his case manager and enjoys the freedom to initiate many of the contacts.

Information sharing
One of the important priorities is for the case manager to communi-cate and demonstrate the difference of the approach to the previously mistrusted contacts with services, in order to build a trusting working relationship. Patrick is a skilled cabinet-maker who feels frustrated by his inability to maintain employment. He takes the opportunity to discuss carpentry skills with the case manager and for them both to consider options that may be available to use his skills outside the pres-sures of the job market. The case manager also offers Patrick and his mother more time to understand and think through what the various offers of support services may entail, both for her physical disability and Patrick's frequent epileptic fits (sometimes necessitating admission to a local A&E department with injuries to head and limbs). Patrick

takes some medication, distrusts changes of medication, yet occasionally self-medicates with alcohol. The case manager offers supportive counselling around the issues.

RISK TAKING

Traditionally mental health services have taken a very cautious approach to the issue of individual service users taking risks of any kind. This is an area of practice where service practitioners tend to be educated, by training and experience, into a paternalistic mould that discourages untested opportunity and leaves the individual service user feeling powerless to change. The notion of a young practitioner making judgements on the ability of an older service user to take responsibility for their actions is yet another grey area of moral and ethical debate. This becomes even more questionable when we consider the frequency with which many practitioners, jokingly or otherwise, quietly question their own abilities to take responsibility for actions governing their own lives!

Bleach (1994) reminds us that there is no current legislation that suggests people experiencing long-term mental health problems have any less of a right to learn from making day-to-day mistakes than anyone else. Most people acknowledge that they learn more from their mistakes, by pushing the boundaries and trying out new challenges. Yet, in the absence of legal powers many practitioners, with the best intentions, resort to a form of 'pestering power' to discourage the individual user from taking a course of action that appears to be 'risky'.

The nature of risk

The retreat to conservatism is understandable in light of the highly publicized traumatic and fatal incidents involving people who have experienced severe mental health problems. It is true that the occasional individual sufferer, through extreme fear and distress, has responded with aggressive actions against others or themselves. It may be argued that an equal tragedy has been allowed through the failure to emphasize the very small proportion of sufferers who reach this point and also the apparent enthusiasm of some to encourage the stigma of mental health by promoting these tragic behaviours as the norm. So the majority of people experiencing mental health difficulties feel even more powerless in the face of unreal expectations that they are all on the brink of axe murders or spectacular suicide plans.

The assessment of risk of harm to self or others is an essential element of the practitioner's responsibility to the individual user, the worker themselves and other colleagues in the network of care and support. Such assessments focus on the negative aspect of risk and as such will be detailed more in Chapter 8. For the purposes of understanding more about the empowering nature of 'risk', we must look more to the positive potentials of risk taking. Hutchinson *et al.* (1990) remind us that some types of risk should be encouraged with the individual user, because this is an essential element of everyday life for all of us.

By far the most empowering aspect of positive risk taking is for the practitioner to let go of the 'professional expert' role and actually ask the service user what it is that they want. They may not always know, partly due to the constant experience of having power removed and being told what is best for them. On these occasions it may be the responsibility of the practitioner to suggest options and to create choices, but definitely not to take the decisions. The least empowering mode of practice would be the all too frequent reliance on the limited psychiatric service options. This approach to positive risk taking will be illuminated further in this chapter under the discussion of the strengths model of case management.

Accommodating 'difference'

Bleach (1994) suggests that genuine attempts to promote user-empowering relationships are reflected in the quality of how we accommodate different standpoints and opinions between the practitioner and the service user. The practitioner and the service user will generally have very different motivations for engaging, or otherwise, in the service that is being offered. Consequently, we have an opportunity to promote a sense of power sharing if we genuinely seek to share and understand these different motivations. The individual is more likely to feel valued and respected if they see the service actively engaging and adapting to their own motivation for seeking the service in the first place.

Similarly the whole area of expectations around what will, what should and what can happen through engaging with a particular service may differ between the prospective service user and the individual practitioner. The individual user may hold expectations of 'cure' or that psychosocial interventions will replace the more common emphasis on medical treatment. Conversely, society's opinion enforced by professional practice may emphasize the issues of 'control' and institutional treatment. Whatever the difference, the individual user may be helped to feel more empowered by receiving full information about the different opinions that may be held.

This brings us back to the most contentious issue of difference, that of the individual user's right to 'refuse' a service. In Chapter 5 we have already discussed the need for creative responses towards a user's right not to engage with a service. These rights should be fully respected, but the individual practitioner is also motivated by the expectation of providing some form of service to a vulnerable person who could be at risk.

The balance of freedom and risk taking can occasionally be a difficult one to achieve.

A problem with this difference of opinion surrounds the dilemma of who is actually making the assessment of vulnerability and on what grounds. Practitioners erring on the side of caution may leave the individual feeling powerless. Second opinions are generally elicited from like-minded professionals, leaving the individual feeling somewhat out-numbered and powerless. There is a role for independent advocates in these situations, provided they carry some recognized power.

The role of advocates will be discussed further in this chapter; however, it still remains vitally important that the individual service user is able to discuss their own reasons for refusing a service and that they are given the full reasons for the practitioner's concerns and assessment of this deci-sion. For the practitioner, respecting the right of refusal becomes easier in the knowledge that other support networks exist to deal with unhealthy elements of risk, should they arise.

Case study 6.2: Edgar (53 years old)

A single man with a 30-year-history of being diagnosed with schizo-phrenia, Edgar experienced long hospital admissions throughout much of the 1960s and 1970s. From 1980 onwards he had a more settled pat-tern of living in a council hostel with only intermittent contact with formal psychiatric services.

'*Difference*'
Edgar denies any experience of psychiatric illness, preferring to explain his circumstances more in terms of his ability to meditate, think on a superior level and his specific interests in philosophy, science and astron-omy. Edgar holds some strong antipsychiatry and antireligious views. He meets the diagnosis of schizophrenia by adopting an interest in the 'nutri-tional' treatments developed through work at Princeton University, USA.

Risk taking
Edgar's variable compliance with psychiatric medication, corresponding with periods of intense staring and occasional mumbling to himself, raises concerns from hostel workers based on their previous experiences of his aggressive outbursts towards other residents. Edgar shares accommodation predominantly with alcohol abusers whom he refers to as 'addicts with inferior intellectual powers'. The potential for inter-personal conflict is constantly high.

Practitioner 'accommodation'
The case manager trades off an acceptance of Edgar's knowledge and opinions about 'nutritional' treatments with encouragement for Edgar to share and discuss this knowledge. Against this, the case manager

gives information to Edgar about the purpose and problems of psychiatric medication. The intended outcome is one of genuinely informed choice.

Information about the strengths approach to case management is presented through acceptance of Edgar's interests and knowledge in philosophy and science. Views and opinions are encouraged for discussion, rather than interpreted as symptoms. The case manager raises the issues around potential for conflict between Edgar and other residents, discussing his assumptions about responsibility (he asserts his neighbours have 'diminished' responsibility for their actions) and what contingency plans he can develop for decreasing the incidence of threats or retreat from potential threats. These discussions include Edgar's perceptions of how he may pose a threat to others by his own presentation of 'difference'.

RIGHTS

An essential aspect of empowering the service user is by providing full and accurate information about their legal and moral rights. Read and Wallcraft (1992, p. 15) sum up this need in their first statement on the checklist of Dos and Don'ts for empowering service users:

> Do let us know what our rights are. Often we feel we have none and are treated as if we have none. Let us know about our rights to refuse treatment, leave, make a complaint or be represented at a mental health tribunal. It helps to be told more than once and to also be given the information in writing.

In addition to some of the rights referred to above, the empowered individual will also be fully informed about such aspects as:

- the choices of care and treatments available;
- access to interpreters, independent advocates, further explanations;
- confidentiality of information and access to medical records;
- rights that still exist when detained under mental health law;
- the terms and labels used around diagnosis and symptomatology;
- the opportunities for a second opinion.

(MIND, 1992b)

THE STRENGTHS APPROACH TO A PRACTICAL PROCESS

The more traditional problem-solving approach adopted by the majority of psychiatric services tends to be service centred in its orientation. It frequently adopts the professional's assessment and prescription of treatment plans, defines the client in terms of their problems and failings, does little for individual empowerment and much more in terms of potential alienation of the individual from the whole process. It is also likely that an approach that focuses on problems will tend to prioritize the medical factors of mental health and medication as the first issues to be resolved, relegating social and environmental issues to a secondary priority, often to be dealt with by someone else.

Beeforth *et al.* (1990) highlight that a good quality empowering service should prioritize the needs and wants expressed by the service user, but not simply limited to the areas of medical expertise, extending acceptance across the wider range of housing, financial, social and daily activity needs.

By contrast to the problem-focused approach, Rapp (1988) suggests that a strengths orientation fosters empowerment through a number of intrinsic factors:

- by promoting partnership in the working relationship;
- by looking for what is 'good' we adopt a positive attitude;
- by seeing possibilities where we previously only saw the limitations;
- by actively sharing and highlighting the positive results.

Furthermore, the strengths approach sets up intentions to promote empowerment by its focus on an outreach perspective. In taking the service to where the client feels more comfortable we are already communicating a wish to share control of the whole process (as outlined in Chapters 3 and 5). Bleach (1994) also highlights the empowering value of taking the process along at the individual service user's pace and respecting their right to withdraw from any particular part of the process if and when they wish.

Engagement

We have already stated the importance of this function in its own right in Chapter 5. It should ideally be addressed before assessment, though in reality the two will intermix to varying degrees depending on the development of the interpersonal relationship. Morgan (1993) suggests that it is important to try and establish similar agendas from the outset. This involves the practitioner becoming involved in the life of the service user, to a certain extent, for the subsequent assessment to be a shared and accurate meaningful task. Bleach (1994) says that such a position may be achieved by the practitioner adopting an unstructured, informal and conversational approach to relax both parties.

Strengths assessment

Kisthardt and Rapp (1989) outline the strengths assessment as a specifically designed tool for helping to present a whole positive personal inventory.

This includes the opportunity to rediscover personal and environmental potentials that may have become clouded or subjugated by the experiences of mental health problems and an oppressive system of care. Bleach (1993) comments that the function of assessment promotes participation through its emphasis on positive strengths, but warns against the disempowering nature of overformal and elaborate paperwork designed to collect details which may be necessary for the service and administration, but which are not necessarily relevant to the process of directly working with the service user.

In order to act as a useful tool within the helping process the strengths assessment should include the following:

- focus on gathering information about the individual's current circumstances, what they want to achieve in the future and what involvements or resources they have used in the past;
- focus on all areas of the individual's life, e.g. housing, finances, health, medication, occupation and leisure, daily living skills, social supports and legal matters;
- be ongoing, because circumstances and desires change, assessment is not static and absolute, new facets of a person continually emerge;
- progress in a simple and informal manner, at a pace that is comfortable for the individual service user;
- be as detailed and specific as possible, in a way that clearly individualizes the person and represents their uniqueness;
- generate a list of the individual's 'wants' rather than the practitioner's list of 'client needs';
- focus on topics that are of interest to the service user, including those that make the process fun for all participants;
- draw up a holistic portrait of the individual;
- provide a logical step on to the development of helping plans.

An example of a strengths assessment is detailed in Table 6.1. It is important to reiterate that the information is largely drawn from the communication between service user and practitioner, based on informal discussions rather than formal interview. The actual paperwork may be presented at individual meetings, depending on the wishes of the individual user, and its completion will be determined entirely by the pace of the discussions, updated as new information arises subsequently. The format is such that it may be completed by:

- the service user, after coaching by the practitioner in the positive orientation of the approach;
- the practitioner, when the service user observes any type of paperwork to be a formality;
- the practitioner outside meetings, where the service user feels alienated by paperwork.

Table 6.1 Case management strengths assessment

Client: Mrs A	Case management	Date: November 1994
Case manager: Steve Morgan	Strengths assessment	
What has worked for me in the *past*?	**What is happening at *present*?**	**What do I want in the *future*?**
	Housing	
Council flats and a women's hostel	One bedroom council flat	'New bricks' with modern and electric central heating
	Financial	
Wages from full and part-time jobs	Income support Disability living allowance Housing benefit Council tax exemption	Stay on social security benefits. 'Turkey money'
	Health	
Hospital admissions. Less activity when I have needed rest to stop me becoming ill	Feeling calm and settled. Not so much stress	To stay out of hospital. Learn to control my own stress levels
	Medication	
Taking tablets and injections sometimes helps me feel settled	Injection at doctor's surgery fortnightly. Tablets every day	Stay the same as long as it keeps me settled
	Occupation and leisure	
Cleaning jobs. Visits to a day hospital	Go to a drop-in centre twice a week. Watch TV for soap operas and horse racing	Do more reading and perhaps a training course in receptionist skills
	Daily living skills	
Doing my own domestic chores and looking after a family. Nigerian cooking	I look after myself, but sometimes have a meal at the drop-in	The pain from disabled wrists to be less, so I can cope better
	Social support	
Having my children at home. Meeting other people at work	Children visit me on weekends. Meet people at the drop-in centre	More contact with Nigerian people, to talk in my own language
	Legal	
Children in Social Services care. Access meetings at the social work office	All children are able to visit at my flat	My daughter to come back to live with me

What's most important for me to do:
1. Stay out of hospital.
2. Move to 'new bricks' (client's term for modern housing).
3. Get my 'turkey money' (client's term for Xmas social security bonus)
4. My daughter to move home with me.

Client signature:	Case manager signature:
Date:	Date:

There is no assumption that the whole of the form has to be completed; parts may be left blank if they are considered irrelevant or confidential for any reason. The format is only truly useful if it is comfortable and acceptable to whoever is compiling the information. However, the holistic positive portrait has proved a valuable exercise and presentable product to the service user who is frequently burdened by their own focus, and that of others, on their failings and inabilities. Frequently, a service user needs to be guided carefully into the approach, because of the intrinsic dominance of distressing experience, though a person's desire to stay with the problems is never diminished or denied by a respecting practitioner.

Strengths care planning

As highlighted in Chapter 3, the care planning function in the strengths case management process is a needs-focused exercise that relates entirely to the assessment of client 'wants'. This is the function of the process where the specific short and longer term goals are detailed in order to follow a path of achievement towards the individual's stated wishes. This may be the point at which it is necessary to detail the problems that could stand in the way of achieving these wishes. Empowerment stems from locating problems in relation to what we desire, rather than the all too familiar situation of targeting problems for their own intrinsic qualities, that require resolution for no greater reason than the problem itself.

Beeforth *et al.* (1994) suggest that in an ideal world service users would be equal partners in the development of the care plan. Kisthardt and Rapp (1989) see the strengths care planning function very much in terms of 'accompanying the client on their journey', by helping to maximize the principle of client self-direction. Bleach (1993) elucidates the partnership in terms of the plans being generated through the perceptions and priorities of the service user, but with the practitioner helping to mediate many external influences on the process, where necessary.

In practical empowering terms the statement of goals in the planning process should be uniquely personalized (Rapp, 1988; Lloyd and Maas, 1992), stated in clearly measurable terms with short-term goals carrying a high probability of success (Kisthardt, 1992). Collecting unnecessary data only confuses the process and alienates the service user (Bleach, 1993). Table 6.2 illustrates an example of strengths care planning.

Monitoring and review

The helping process is a cyclical format, moved on and informed by a regular period of review. Kisthardt (1992) suggests this is a collective function, but to be empowering it needs to be fully shared and owned by

Table 6.2 Case management strengths personal plan

Client: Mrs A	Case management	Date: November 1994
Case manager: Steve Morgan	Strengths personal plan	

Client goal: **To stay out of hospital**

Medium-term goals	**Responsibility**
1. Regular monitoring of health	Mrs A & S. Morgan
2. Attending outpatient appointments	Mrs A

Short-term goals	**Responsibility**
1. Identify three early warning signs of stress	Mrs A & S. Morgan
2. Reduce activity levels immediately when feeling tired or stressed	Mrs A
3. Regular attendance at GP surgery for injections fortnightly	Mrs A

Client goal: **To move to new bricks**

Medium-term goals	**Responsibility**
1. Complete council housing transfer application	Mrs A
2. Complete medical application	Mrs A

Short-term goals	**Responsibility**
1. Collect application forms from local housing office	Mrs A
2. Discuss reasons for move and the supportive medical information	Mrs A & S. Morgan
3. Complete application and place it with local housing office	Mrs A & S. Morgan

Client signature:	Case manager signature:	Review date: March 1995

the service user, targeting progress in relation to their goals and desires. Furthermore, it is important that all successes, however small they may first appear, should be clearly recognized and reinforced. The collective function may be initiated through user involvement in setting the agenda for the review meeting.

Read and Wallcraft (1992) include the following characteristics of a 'good' review meeting, from the service user's perspective:

- access to the support of an independent advocate or trusted friend at the meeting;
- to have a say in who is invited and where it may be held;
- a keyworker should be responsible for regular liaison with the service user and the advocate;
- the fewer people in attendance, the less daunting it may be;

- avoid use of jargon, but offer clear explanations;
- the service user's questions should be answered and opinions respected as the most central to the discussion;
- an opportunity should be offered after the meeting for discussion of feelings with the keyworker and/or advocate.

Furthermore, any disagreement expressed by the service user should be equally minuted in the report of the meeting.

Users' evaluation of the process

From the professional's viewpoint some fairly strong user-empowering claims have been made for the process, including that the respective roles of professional and client have dramatically changed with the user encouraged to adopt more control of the decision-making process. Also that the very language of the approach belongs to the client (Weick *et al.*, 1989). Only service users themselves can truly say whether such claims are met or exaggerated.

The work of Beeforth *et al.* (1994) was a genuinely independent user evaluation of the Sainsbury Centre for Mental Health case management project, a project that widely adopted aspects of the strengths approach. Among its findings, this evaluation has found the accessibility and relationship orientation of the approach to promote a much greater user involvement in decision making. This was despite initial assumptions that case management may be potentially 'controlling' in its all-encompassing service role. Greater control in decisions also leads onto greater user control over subsequent plans and actions, with an overall empowering feeling and greater individual self-esteem.

On the other hand, case management was found to have little or no impact on areas of resource deficiencies, particularly failing to impact on opportunities for returning to paid employment. The evaluation also unearthed some continuing dissatisfaction with the continued use of hospitalizations with little creative searching for community alternatives and many issues around the prescription and administration of medications still left service users feeling disempowered.

BOUNDARIES

The potential intensity and encompassing nature of the working relationship poses a dilemma in terms of establishing boundaries. The case management relationship is occasionally criticized by other professionals for its potential blurring of roles between what can clearly be delineated as 'professional' and that which becomes friendship. Conversely, many service users criticize the practitioner for adopting the formality of professionalism, when what they would value more highly is a degree of friendship in the relationship. The balance is a difficult one to set guidelines for. Once again it requires sensitivity to individual circumstances and a careful guarding against becoming overfriendly, when it no longer feels comfortable expressing objective views for fear of losing some of the familiarity and friendship. At this point, the potential for a constructive working relationship is passed by and the worker is just as likely to give out their own telephone number and address and make regular visits out of working hours.

It is important to develop an early understanding of the type of limits and boundaries that may be established, that hold two people to a working relationship without denying some of the informality that is more characteristic of friendship. This issue closely reflects that of 'self-disclosure' outlined in Chapter 4. Certain degrees of self-disclosure help to establish a positive atmosphere of trust, by enabling a service user to work with a person rather than a professional title.

ADVOCACY ROLES

In respect of the case management relationship, Witheridge (1989) suggests that a great deal of the practitioner's time is spent acting as an advocate for service users who find themselves in conflict with complex and impersonal bureaucracies on which they depend for much needed help. Kanter (1989) elucidates this role further as the ability to articulate the client's needs to provider agencies, empathize with the concerns and priorities of the providers and then maintain a position of ongoing dialogue whilst supporting the client. This latter point introduces the common dilemma of professionals and advocacy roles. While the service provider would prefer to advocate for the client's stated wishes, their professional status frequently leads them to prioritize their own assessment of the client's best interests.

It is frequently found that a professional is able to accommodate strong advocacy roles in the area of work that do not impinge on their own contract of employment. For example, a health worker will be more free to advocate in areas such as housing and social security, but feel more restricted in advocating health needs that conflict with professional judgement. The ability to empower individual user's through advocacy roles is therefore limited. In these instances, it is much more valuable and empowering if the service practitioner feels able to access independent self, citizen or legal advocates, as the need arises. For the practitioner, a balance needs to be struck between the more ideal use of independent advocates for all advocacy roles and the important relationship-enhancing function that can be harnessed by the practitioner successfully advocating for some user needs.

EMPOWERMENT OR DEPENDENCY

Harris (1990) suggests that case managers constantly confront the issue of how to provide a wide-ranging supportive service without creating an inevitable dependency by the user on the practitioner. Dangers are foreseen equally in the circumstances where the relationship creates over- or underexpectations and it is the service user who will ultimately feel disempowered by the failure at either extreme.

It is often assumed that practitioners will err on the side of underachievement, but Wills (1982) reminds us that encouraging greater user-led control can have positive rewards in practice, rather than be threatening to helpers themselves. Staff have to work within constraints set by their employers, so the argument may often follow the lines of 'I would if I could, but ... '. Read and Wallcraft (1992) argue that even within employer parameters, there are still choices that can be made by the individual practitioner which clearly indicate whether they favour degrees of empowerment or paternalism. 'No-one can give power to another person, but they can stop taking their power away. They can also help people to regain their own power, ... ' (Read and Wallcraft, 1992, p. 5).

SUMMARY

This chapter has essentially attempted to discuss how the individual relationship between a service provider and a service user can help the latter to take a more prominent role in determining the nature and direction of their own needs for care and support. The issues are those of exercising the power of choice and decision making about your own life. Barker and Peck (1987) draw an analogy with 'travel' when they suggest that empowerment is as much about the 'journey' of attitude changes that practitioners and users have to adapt as it is about the 'destination' of service outcomes for the individual user. Empowment has to be experienced rather than legislated for or imposed.

The reason we all need to give special consideration to the subject of empowerment is referred to by Rogers *et al.* (1993) when they ask how acceptable mental health services have been to their users. They rightly imply that the necessity and helpfulness of traditional psychiatric services, assumed by the professionals, are greatly overrated when we consider the amount of pestering and coercion that seems to be involved, even with informal users.

Service users have widely upheld informality and flexibility as essential characteristics of the voluntary sector provisions (Rogers *et al.*, 1993) and case management services (Beeforth *et al.*, 1994), in contrast to the more structured hierarchical development of traditional statutory sector services. A more empowering, user-led service would prioritize voluntary relationships rather than coercion, user participation and leadership roles, self-advocacy, self-help groups and favours social over medical needs (Rogers *et al.*, 1993).

However, these empowering alternatives do not carry the assumption that professional skills become redundant, but rather than practitioners need to use their skills in different ways, through listening and attending, supporting user priorities and promoting choices. Finally, Read and Wallcraft (1992, p. 15) advise us: 'Don't hide behind a mask of professionalism. Don't use words we don't understand. Don't pretend you know more than you do. Mental health work is full of uncertainty, confusion, controversy and contradictions. Honesty is empowering'.

REFERENCES

Barker, I. and Peck, E. (eds) (1987) *Power in Strange Places*, Good Practices in Mental Health, London.

Beeforth, M., Conlan, E., Field, V. *et al.* (1990) *Whose Service is it Anyway?* Research and Development for Psychiatry, London.

Beeforth, M., Conlan, E. and Graley, R. (1994) *Have We Got Views For You: User Evaluation of Case Management*, Sainsbury Centre for Mental Health, London.

Bleach, A. (1993) Top of the form. *Community Care*, 23rd September, 24–5.

Bleach, A. (1994) *'Engagement' Draft Training Module*, Sainsbury Centre for Mental Health, London.

Chamberlain, J. (1988) *On Our Own*, MIND, London.

Harris, M. (1990) Redesigning case management services for work with character-disordered young adult patients, in *Psychiatry Takes to the Streets,* (ed. N.L. Cohen), The Guilford Press, New York, pp. 156–76.

Hutchinson, M., Linton, G. and Lucas, J. (1990) *User Information Pack: From Policy to Practice*, MIND South East, London.

Kanter, J. (1989) Clinical case management: definition, principles, components. *Hospital and Community Psychiatry*, **40**(4), 361–8.

Kisthardt, W.E. (1992) A strengths model of case management: the principles and functions of a helping partnership with persons with persistent mental illness, in *A Strengths Perspective for Social Work Practice*, (ed. D. Saleeby), Longman, New York, pp. 59–83.

Kisthardt, W.E. and Rapp, C.A. (1989) *Bridging the Gap Between Principles and Practice: Implementing a Strengths Perspective in Case Management*, University of Kansas, Lawrence.

Lloyd, C. and Maas, F. (1992) Interpersonal skills and occupational therapy. *British Journal of Occupational Therapy*, **55**(10), 379–82.

MIND (1992a) *The MIND Guide to Advocacy in Mental Health: Empowerment in Action*, MIND, London.

MIND (1992b) *Being Informed and Giving Consent: A Checklist for Users of Mental Health Services*, MIND, London.

Morgan, S. (1993) *Community Mental Health: Practical Approaches to Long-Term Problems*, Chapman & Hall, London.

Rapp, C.A. (1988) *The Strengths Perspective of Case Management with Persons Suffering from Severe Mental Illness*, NIMH and University of Kansas, Lawrence.

Read, J. and Wallcraft, J. (1992) *Guidelines for Empowering Users of Mental Health Services*, MIND and COHSE, London.

Rogers, A., Pilgrim, D. and Lacey, R. (1993) *Experiencing Psychiatry: User's Views of Services*, Macmillan, London.

Stewart, A. (1994) Empowerment and enablement: occupational therapy 2001. *British Journal of Occupational Therapy*, **57**(7) 248–54.

Weick, A., Rapp, C., Sullivan, W.P. and Kisthardt, W.E. (1989) A strengths perspective for social work practice. *Social Work*, **33**, 350–4.

Wills, T.A. (ed.) (1982) *Basic Processes in Helping Relationships*, Academic Press, New York.

Witheridge, T.F. (1989) The assertive community treatment worker: an emerging role and its implications for professional training. *Hospital and Community Psychiatry*, **40**(6), 620–4.

FURTHER READING

Leiper, R. and Field, V. (eds) (1993) *Counting for Something*, Avebury, London.

Lindow, V. (1994) *Self Help Alternatives to Mental Health Services*, MIND, London.

McIver, S. (1991) *Obtaining the Views of Users of Mental Health Services*, King's Fund Centre, London.

Rogers, A. and Pilgrim, D. (1991) Pulling down churches: accounting for the British mental health users movement. *Sociology of Health and Illness*, **13**(2), 129–48.

Sociocultural considerations | 7

Since psychiatric practices have historically developed in a predominantly Western cultural framework, largely through the leadership of
white, middle-class males, we need to recognize the very strong social
pressures and political issues that will impinge on all people involved,
users and practitioners (Fernando, 1988). The emergence of multiracial
and multicultural communities and the recognition of the need to
accept greater gender equality mean that a range of hitherto neglected
sociocultural considerations will now affect the development of individual relationships. Innate, conscious or subconscious racist and
sexist values only serve to diminish the quality of such a working
relationship.

As we have seen from the discussion in Chapter 6, 'power' is a major
factor in many aspects of interpersonal relationships, exercised through
values, attitudes, beliefs and even the terminology we adopt. The predominance of male characteristics as the baseline for psychiatric research
has been challenged (Bachrach and Nadelson, 1988) and clearly the use
of terms such as 'minority' in relation to ethnic groups is charged with
overt power differentials (d'Ardenne and Mahtani, 1989).

Power is frequently exercised at a collective group level, intrinsically
becoming a sociopolitical issue, but in this chapter we will highlight how
it is also exercised actually or potentially at the individual level. It is
frequently seen in the stereotyping of diagnosis on the basis of flawed
observation of behaviours rather than feelings (Brand and McGinley,
1986) and the way behaviour can be influenced by the structure and
design of so many clinical settings. It is also seen in the way some studies
and research methods assume from the outset that the causes of illness
must be within individuals rather than in the social conditions they have
to experience (Gobodo, 1992).

This chapter will focus particularly on the issues of race, culture and gender, how these sociopolitical issues impinge on the individual user and practitioner relationship and what constitutes good supportive and interactive practice. Other considerations, such as sexual orientation, social class, age and religious beliefs, are equally central to discriminatory practices but may only be referred to in a peripheral manner here, so I apologize to any reader who feels their specific interests have been excluded.

RACE AND CULTURE

These two terms are frequently intermixed and confused, unintentionally or otherwise. Fernando (1988) suggests that social anthropologists have initiated this confusion by the assertion that if an individual originates from a particular 'race' they will exhibit the 'cultural' traits identifiable to that race. Predominantly white psychiatric practitioners have adopted this confusion in a way that promotes ideas of 'cultural' understanding as a cover for what is often an underlying racial issue. Dominelli (1988) suggests that such an understanding of cultural difference acts as a barrier to tackling real racist practices.

The inference from the ongoing development of this confusion is that 'culture', with its wide diversity of meaning, is easier to discuss and perhaps a more acceptable concept in psychiatry than the more politically charged 'race'. For similar reasons, the term 'ethnic' is frequently substituted for race. The fear seems to arise from the difficulty of separating the concept of race from charges of racism in psychiatric practice, so this is somehow diluted by the replacement with apparently more neutral terminology.

It appears that the early discussions of the differences between whites and blacks focused more on racial superiority and inferiority, with no particular reference to cultural context. The white Anglo-Saxon saw race as a biological concept, with black people being inferior on a number of apparent biological comparisons (Fernando, 1988). The perpetuation of such myths form the basis of racism but despite a growing understanding that race is about more than biological differences, including a combination of social, political and cultural factors, the inherent oppression of individuals and groups necessitates that racist practices demand more attention than the theoretical concept of race.

The concepts of race and culture do overlap significantly, but in order to fathom out some of the confusion we need to firstly separate out that which can be more clearly defined.

Racism

Lorde defines racism as '... the belief in the inherent superiority of one race over all others and thereby the right to dominance' (1984, p. 115). Racism can be subdivided into types and Dominelli (1989) refers to the following categorization:

- individual racism; personal attitudes and behaviour that are used to prejudge racial groups negatively;
- institutional racism; public legitimation of prejudice, including the power of exclusion used against apparently inferior groups;
- cultural racism; values, beliefs and ideas which endorse the superiority of white culture.

The broad impact of institutional racism on its individual victim is the potential of poor educational opportunities, poor expectations, poor job opportunities and various forms of social stereotyping. The reality of racist practices in the institution of psychiatry will not be so different from the racism the individual may experience from the other 'institutions', e.g. judiciary or police.

In terms of racial stereotypes, Fernando quotes a Brent Community Health Council report, which states: 'In the National Health Service the mythology is that Afro-Caribbean women are feckless and irresponsible, while Asian women are compliant but stupid. West Indians are dubbed as having no culture, the problem for Asians *is* their culture' (Fernando, 1988, p. 56). Consequently, many members of different ethnic groups who enter the psychiatric system find themselves having to cope with the prejudice described above, combined with an institutionalized fear of black people by white people, which then permeates the attitudes towards diagnosis and treatment. Brand and McGinley (1986) state that a member of a different racial group is likely to receive higher amounts of psychotropic drugs in order to control behaviours, less access to the psychotherapeutic treatments due to a lack of understanding of psycho-dynamic factors that are culturally based and a higher risk of detention in the more punitive facilities.

Lewisham, in South-East London, has made some progressive efforts in the statutory and voluntary sectors to make services more racially and culturally aware. However, these initiatives need to be viewed against a background of the following statements:

- 24% of the total population are 'black' people;
- black users are overrepresented in the mental health services at over double their representation in the local population;
- 50–80% of users of acute psychiatric services are 'black' people;
- black users and carers have reported being unsatisfied with the services they received;
- staff report being unaware of and untrained in the racial and cultural backgrounds of many of their service users.

In response to some of these initial findings the Guy's and Lewisham NHS Trust Mental Health Unit (1992) prepared a code of practice which listed the following examples of discrimination to improve the level of staff awareness and sensitivity:

Direct discrimination
a) It is discriminatory to carry out routine urine and blood screening of black clients for drugs simply on the belief that drug abuse is prevalent in the black community; clinical evidence is required to be demonstrated before use of screening on any individual regardless of race.
b) Decisions on the management of potential violence should not be made on assumptions about factors to do with skin colour, physical appearance or physique.
c) Routine prescription of PRN medication for black clients, simply on the assumption they might be dangerous, is discriminating.
d) The use of family or friends as interpreters of 'rights' and 'care plans' simply because of convenience is discriminatory.
e) The allocation of keyworkers should be based on clinical judgements, not the discriminatory demands of staff *or* clients.

Indirect discrimination
a) The provision of written information in the language of some clients, but not that of other identified people.
b) Failing to cater for particular dietary needs.
c) Poor provisions for or neglect of non-Christian religious observance.
d) The provision of reminiscence and social groups for the indigenous population.

These examples are only a guide, not an exhaustive list.

Fernando (1988) suggests that racist values and practices have infiltrated psychiatry in many ways, not just in the training and experience of its individual practitioners but also in the research methods and observations. The result is that the stereotypes based on racist assumptions become incorporated into its research to provide self-fulfilling prophecies. Furthermore, there tends to be a widespread resistance among practitioners to even examining their own racist practices. One example of the mechanisms of racism would be the common misunderstanding by white people of common characteristics of black people, e.g. their tendency to often be more spontaneously vocal, direct and more exuberant in tone and mannerisms. Misunderstanding leads to attempts to control such behaviours, leading to a reaction of outrage, which in itself underpins misdiagnosis.

In relation to the question of misdiagnosis, much discussion has focused on the overrepresentation of black people diagnosed with schizophrenia and held under section of the Mental Health Act or in secure units. However, Eleftheriadou (1994) also suggests a more recent trend of misdiagnosis in relation to social class; black people of relatively low social status are more frequently diagnosed with schizophrenia, whereas black people of higher social status are more frequently diagnosed with manic depression.

Dominelli (1989) outlines a list of strategies that are often adopted to deny or diminish the acknowledgement of racism:

- decontextualization: acknowledge racism in general terms, but not in daily interactions;
- denial: prejudice may occur in some individuals, but not at the institutional or cultural levels;
- colour-blind: suggesting that all people are essentially the same;
- patronizing: a false acceptance of equality;
- omission: racism is not an important part of social interaction;
- avoidance: accept the existence of racism, but deny any personal responsibility for action;
- dumping: responsibility for eliminating racism is placed with 'black workers'.

At the individual working relationship level, Dominelli (1989) further warns us of the dangers of professionalizing the interactions into some form of one-to-one vacuum, isolating the possible impacts of racism out of the priorities to be worked on. This situation reflects the decontextualization strategies mentioned above, whereby the service user becomes an individual person but not necessarily an individual 'black' person. The danger is that we overlook or blatantly ignore much of the uniqueness of the person and we also set up the potential for avoiding many of the problems and potentials that the social environment burdens the individual with.

Case study 7.1: Peter (39 years old)

A man of Afro-Caribbean origin who has lived alone in a succession of council flats since his separation and divorce ten years ago. Contact with psychiatric services inpatient units has been on three occasions via the legal system charged for theft, possession of illegal drugs and indecent exposure. Peter vigorously denies the need for psychiatric medication, admits regular use of cannabis and other unspecified illegal drugs, neglects his personal appearance and that of his flat (through personal admission), avoids payment of bills, always with an intention of paying later, and states that he prefers the drop-in style of 'homeless' facilities to that of organized mental health day care.

Housing

Peter has at one time been placed in a hard-to-let flat in a known racist area of London, on an estate with a high level of drug-related problems. He was the victim of persistent racial harassment and thefts, going to extraordinary lengths of depriving himself of home furnishings in the hope of reducing the purpose for attacks. Despite the council's race assessment unit giving him a high priority for quick housing transfer, the housing office managed to 'administrate' this status away with little logical explanation. Despite full knowledge of his predicament and occasional requests for increased police patrols it was a full 12 months after the 'racial harassment' priority before Peter was finally transferred.

Health

Peter has had repeated confidential assessments of danger, all declaring the need for extreme caution on behalf of staff. He has been banned from one day centre for suspected theft and 'threatening behaviours' of an unspecified nature. He continues to be visited by two members of staff on each occasion. He has been known to collect knives, though he will always give explanations for his own need and use of them. A healthy level of staff caution should be exercised working with all clients, but more attention needs to be paid to the degree of assessment that is made on bizarre personal neglect and on assumptions around skin colour and drug abuse.

Culture

As a term, 'culture' is widely used in common everyday language, but the diversity of its use makes it very difficult to pin down to any precise definition. Anthropologists, politicians, psychiatrists and others use the term to suit their own particular purpose. For some people it refers to everyday activities as well as conceptual ideologies. Some definitions include physical elements of road layouts, building construction and methods as elements that uphold the difference between societies. For others, it is the more subjective aspects of beliefs, myths, values and attitudes that provide the essential differences of cultures.

D'Ardenne and Mahtani (1989) suggest that in the common use of the term, culture can be considered to mean any difference that is identified between one group of people and another. Their succinct but broad-ranging definition states that culture is: 'the shared history, practices, beliefs and values of a racial, regional or religious group of people' (p. 4). Within the broad definition we can identify some of the physical elements mentioned above, that are identified by aspects of design, and also many of the non-material aspects of shared experience such as family systems, childrearing practices, respect for elders, ethical values, common behaviours and cognitions that relate to beliefs, feelings and adaptation to external influences (Fernando, 1988).

If we consider the cultural responses to health in general and psychiatry in particular, we find at the broadest level that Western and non-Western cultures view the concepts of health, illness and medical practice in quite different ways. The integration or division of psychological and physical aspects of health can have considerable cultural implications. However, we are not just referring here to the societal level; it is equally important at the individual practitioner–service user relationship level for the practitioner to understand the user's cultural viewpoints on illness, treatment, healing or faith healing. The individual user may hold quite different but equally valid views on the experience of symptomatology. Different cultures may also promote very different behavioural reactions to such experiences as stress and bereavement, which the Western practitioner may be quick to interpret as symptoms of psychotic illness.

Fernando (1988) suggests that being 'culturally sensitive' is not enough. We need to have a greater understanding of the way people think of and react to illness, for without this understanding the development of individual working relationships will be poor or superficial at best. We need to be sensitive to the reasons why some people experiencing mental health problems become isolated from their own cultural community or in extreme circumstances may even deny their cultural identity, due to the potential stigma of mental illness. Furthermore, we need to acknowledge the complications experienced by people of second or third generations who are born in the UK and attempt to slowly pace their cultural self-discovery. People of mixed race face similarly complex issues of cultural identity, in the face of very stigmatizing opinions held in society.

Finally, d'Ardenne and Mahtani (1989) note that some of the more emotive aspects of culture, namely 'race' and 'class', are often avoided because of their ability to confront people with their own deeply held prejudices. We are reminded that the very process of observing and defining the culture of another person cannot happen in isolation from our own cultural identity. We define culture in terms relative to our own experience; therefore, we need to be more aware of our own cultural inheritance and identity, including how we attempt to modify or adjust our ideas on race. Whilst the white person's view of race originated in the apparent identification of biological and genetic difference, largely by skin colour, our knowledge and experience from multiracial and multicultural societies suggest that these differences should be observed without prejudice. Race is less of an issue of biology and genetics and more to do with social, political and cultural factors (Reber, 1985).

Issues of communication

Within the context of the individual relationship I wish to outline three important issues of communication that may significantly influence the quality of contact between two people of different racial and cultural backgrounds. The first is the use of language, which leads on to the potential uses of interpreters and finally, the issue of underused psychotherapeutic and counselling skills with people of different origins.

Language

Language is a central feature of communication between two people, though the trained observer will be aware that the non-verbal forms of body language are often more significant than the verbal, if interpreted correctly. The language of racial and cultural contexts can be both highly emotive and confused. D'Ardenne and Mahtani (1989) suggest that terms such as 'ethnic' should more clearly belong to 'cultural' vocabulary and 'black' has more of an identification with the discussion of 'racism'. It is important to consider how easily we may misuse or misinterpret phrases differently from the person sharing the working relationship, as trust and confidence in the practitioner could quite easily hinge on their use of words.

A race and culture awareness training session organized by Lewisham and Guy's Mental Health NHS Trust used for its introduction a number of questions for each individual to consider, based around the use of terminology. Some are questions and some are statements, but I will leave you to consider your own personal, possibly cultural, response.

1. 'Immigrants' – most immigrants in the UK are white people; most black people in the UK are not.
2. 'Black' – are Asian people 'black' and if so, in what context?
3. 'Asians' – the many peoples across the Asian continent are not homogeneous in cultural origin.
4. 'Caribbeans' – Indian subcontinent, Chinese and white populations are of significant numbers in the Caribbean islands.
5. 'Indigenous'
   'Host'   } Do these terms have a standard meaning to
   'Second generation'   all people?

The TULIP Outreach and Development Service, in north London, have developed some clear guidelines for what they consider to be 'acceptable' and 'accessible' language in the development of the working relationship. In terms of 'acceptable' language, 'black and minority ethnic people' is used, though we have already established that 'minority' carries connotations of marginalizing people and highlighting powerlessness (d'Ardenne and Mahtani, 1989). Primarily, individuals should be encouraged to be self-defining, with the practitioner adopting sufficient flexibility to accept each person's own definition. In this way, a service user is free to use terms such as Asian, Somali, African-Caribbean, Trinidadian, as they feel best fits their own assumptions of ethnic origin. The TULIP organization also highlights the need to avoid stereotypical terms, e.g. Arabs in place of country of origin, unless this is checked out as suitable to the individual. Most importantly, the service practitioner needs to be aware of the need to adopt language that gives dignity and respect to the service user.

'Accessible' language is that which is jargon-free, available in written form in many different translations to meet the needs of the locally identified populations, with access to interpreters and/or repeated clearer messages to facilitate understanding.

The issue of language difference has resulted in some black people learning to relate to white professionals via a 'proxy self', whereby they attempt to fit in with white expectations of them. However, such a situation does very little to foster a genuine therapeutic alliance or working relationship. Issues of interpreting ideas through language can form the basis of power and control, particularly where practitioners are seen to hide behind professional boundaries.

A further source of misunderstanding and power differential lies in the breaking down of concepts into their simpler descriptive terms. White professionals can address white clients with a wider range of terminology through more simplified language to explain what they mean; however, neither person possesses the same flexibility and quantity of language to afford clearer explanations when the white professional engages with a black client.

Fernando (1988) suggests that while language is a vital part of establishing good rapport in a relationship, other qualities in the practitioner may occasionally be more important, such as empathy, sympathy, humility and an openness to learn from the knowledge and experience of the service user.

Case study 7.2: Edwin and Catherine (61 and 57 years old)

A married couple both originating from Jamaica and living in England for almost 30 years. Edwin had a long-standing diagnosis of schizophrenia and had been considered to have a mild learning disability. His strong accent, combined with frequent outbursts of anger associated with persistent experiences of frightening persecutory feelings, made it difficult for most people to understand what he was saying. Catherine had suffered a severe stroke, which caused her to slur her speech.

Both Edwin and Catherine were dependent on each other for different types of support, so much so that they were generally welcoming to visitors to their flat but resistant to offers of help that may undermine their joint feeling of independence. For a white male worker the temptation would be to make a thorough medical and functional assessment (without necessarily a complete understanding of verbal communications), offer support services and suggest a cultural element through knowledge of locally available culturally organized and/or sensitive services. Such an approach had previously rightly been dismissed by Edwin and Catherine and would reasonably have been dismissed again, whatever the good intentions that may underlie any recommendations.

The more acceptable approach involved the case manager adopting a more open befriending function, getting to know Edwin and Catherine over a protracted period of time, always respectful of their wishes, open to learning from them about their origins and cultural expectations. The initial language barrier was accepted on both sides, with the case manager requesting permission to repeat questions and check out his understanding in a respectful manner. Adopting some of Edwin and Catherine's use of terminology and a degree of practitioner self-disclosure about his young family also helped to establish a friendly rapport.

Ultimately, the case manager was able to introduce areas of service provision that proved acceptable, withdraw any suggestions that were unacceptable and use the relationship with the couple to inform, educate, interpret information, but always to be open to learn from them about their own ideas, wishes and experiences. The bond became significant enough that offers of 'black' or 'African-Caribbean' workers were rejected by Edwin and Catherine, their justification being that it is the person and their personal approach that matters more than the colour of their skin.

Edwin ultimately contracted a terminal illness; he and Catherine chose to request more intensive supportive contact from the white worker throughout this most difficult of experiences.

Use of interpreters

Occasionally the language barrier is insurmountable, whatever the personal qualities of the individuals involved, and there is a need for an interpreter to aid the two-way communication. Fernando (1988) reminds us that at this point it becomes a three-way communication, as information filters in two languages through a third person. D'Ardenne and Mahtani (1989) indicate that the right of all people to understand and be understood is quite 'radical', particularly as many white people believe it is the responsibility of the other person to learn the language if they wish to make full use of services in the UK.

Access to and use of interpreters can be problematic, as outlined in detail by Shackman (1985). Problems can arise around the expectations of control during the interview where an interpreter is being used, but also around the status of the interpreter. On one occasion an official interpreter had been requested by staff of an inner London teaching hospital, only to find that the person sent was the brother of the particular patient and also a previous inpatient of the psychiatric services himself. Confidentiality and the dynamics of interpreting symptomatology and personal experiences were declared to be impossible in the particular circumstances.

Family members or friends have all too frequently been used, on the basis of convenience, as interpreters. This is a particularly unsatisfactory practice when we consider the sensitivity and emotional content of some issues that frequently need to be discussed. Even when official interpreters are available, we need to be accurate about the match of languages, dialects and cultures. A further example in inner London was the use of a member of a Vietnamese mental health association as an interpreter for a client who had arrived from Vietnam but spoke no English. The North–South divide in Vietnam had been overlooked with the consequence that the client refused to speak with the proposed interpreter.

A few guidelines may help the establishing of a relationship through the use of interpreters:

- Hold a preinterview meeting with the interpreter to find ways of assessing potential difference with the client and to ensure role clarity.
- Be assertive with other relatives or friends who may wish to interfere with the course of the interview, giving their own opinions.
- Ensure word-for-word translation, where possible.
- If family members must be used, check out the potential to eliminate difficult or embarrassing concepts, e.g. children translating personal and sexual relationships of a parent.

Psychotherapeutic approaches

Such approaches are culturally rooted in Western societies and are based on communication between a therapist and a client. It may be assumed that significant differences in life experiences and cultural background will present a barrier to the quality of the communication and this is commonly held as a reason why members of different racial and cultural groups are underrepresented in terms of referral for psychotherapeutic treatments.

To be successful the treatment method should hold some resonance with the basic philosophy of the client. Even if they share a common language, there may be significant differences of attitude towards self-disclosure of some issues, interaction in groups, the hierarchical or equal basis of the relationship. Fernando (1988) suggests that in many cases the essential elements of communication and rapport, interest in client feelings and supportive actions in response to feelings should be adapted to other cultural expectations by a flexible practitioner.

Practitioner self-awareness

One of the difficulties already alluded to in this chapter has been the question of white practitioners assessing their own racist practices that come from their own cultural origins, training and experience in a predominantly white, middle-class system of healthcare. In order to become more 'culturally sensitive', practitioners need to become more aware of the influence their own culture has on attitudes and clinical judgements; self-awareness becomes a precursor to improved awareness of others (Bavington and Majid, 1986). Fernando (1988) suggests that 'culture sensitivity' through self-awareness and openness to experience is as useful as any specific training that may be organized.

D'Ardenne and Mahtani (1989) indicate that self-awareness comes from attention to a number of sources:
- personal experiences and information, from reading, travel or living in a multicultural neighbourhood;
- personal and institutional resources, including family, social networks, religious beliefs, personal healthcare, political beliefs, training, education and employment history;
- personal attitudes and expectations towards ideas and experiences of 'difference'; racist practices can be quite subtle and subconscious;
- personal development and application of counselling skills;
- personal perceptions of status as a practitioner.

Relationship skills

Rapport

The starting point for developing rapport will always be the context in which the initial meeting takes place. An outreach perspective will be valued by some as respecting their desire to avoid the institutional service settings that they perceive to be racially and culturally threatening. However, other people set a higher priority on the potential invasion of their own personal space. If the service user perceives the consultation to be enforced, it is more likely to take on a context of social control by the 'system'. Conversely, if a greater element of choice is introduced, rapport may be determined more by client perceptions of the individual practitioner.

Sources of failure to achieve rapport may focus on user perceptions of the individual practitioner as an agent of the system. This may arise particularly where the service provider is seen to dogmatically hold to institutional perceptions of psychiatric diagnosis, assessment interpretations and priorities for treatment.

Trust

In the context of racial and cultural working relationships, the development of trust needs to overcome more than the simple question of care and support. Fernando (1988) suggests that many clients will intrinsically see the practitioner as the representative of a system that perpetuates racial and cultural biases. Even 'black' workers have to overcome the suspicion of black clients that they simply represent a 'white' system. Trust may be initiated if the practitioner can demonstrate some form of loosening of the tie between themselves and the institution and place the emphasis more on the personal relationship with the client. Demonstrating a personal sensitivity to race, culture and the circumstances of the individual may help to initiate trust. This may be seen as a degree of self-disclosure, which Sue and Sue (1990) suggest is an important aspect of trustworthiness if it is honest, open and appropriate to the situation.

Empathy

Gobodo (1992) notes that it is often not so much the differences between two people that influence the ability to communicate empathy but the practitioner's attitudes towards accepting and respecting those differences. We outlined the concept of empathy in Chapter 4; if we accept that it is a way of 'being with' the client, then we need to pay particular attention to culturally different responses towards the helping process. One such difference may be a focus on practical problems in the present, rather than the psychotherapeutic focus on the influence of historical development. Some clients also come to the relationship seeking direct advice and problem solving, which may be in initial conflict with a non-directive, client-centred approach as illustrated in this text by the strengths case management approach.

Empathy is also very much about communicating back the practitioner's understanding of the client's experience. Some people require more direct information, which has been an issue for some commentators; Brand and McGinley (1986) have particularly noted how service providers have frequently treated black clients and carers as 'stupid', by the lack of information that is passed on. Clearly there has been little empathic understanding of needs, let alone abilities.

Case study 7.3: Mr MAT (46 years old)

Mr MAT is of Ugandan-Asian origin, arriving in the UK in the early 1970s with his parents and siblings, as a part of the large migration out of Uganda at the time. He has been diagnosed with schizophrenia for nearly 15 years, has experienced a 20-year history of alcohol abuse and made several serious suicide attempts in response to depressive episodes combined with derogatory hallucinatory voices.

Mr MAT has lived alone for much of the time since he left the family home 12 years ago; due to his alcohol abuse the strictly Moslem family have tended to feel exasperated by his behaviours in the face of their attempts to support him. The statutory services, through a case management approach, had helped him to achieve some success with periods of abstinence and his family have agreed to a partnership of support with the case manager.

Mr MAT's elderly father frequently sleeps at his flat and accompanies him to most new plans that he agrees to try. Mr MAT's stated priorities are to stop drinking alcohol and to achieve a 'more settled and peaceful life'.

Cultural considerations
The first consideration for the case manager was to enquire of the client what name he preferred to be addressed by. He chose M, though other services had referred to him variously as A, T or Mr AT. His family refer to him as A, a name passed to males through the family generations.

Mr T Snr, the elderly father, influenced by the protracted alcohol abuse of his son, felt the only solution would be for his son to be accompanied in activity every waking hour. Mr MAT wished to achieve a combination of support and trusting independence. The case manager was required to negotiate an acceptable compromise between Mr MAT's personal dilemma of how to manage his own balance between Moslem traditions and British traditions, with his father's stronger Moslem traditions and concern for his son's health.

Mr T Snr feels a need to 'check out' the credentials of any new workers that become involved in his son's care, with concern for the cultural acceptance of the approaches, as well as an intention to establish his own supportive presence for his son.

Mr MAT has experienced his first full involvement in the holy month of Ramadan, without the distraction of alcohol, for many years. Whilst the family felt an extra reason for 'celebration', Mr MAT became confused as to how he could continue his prescribed medication. The case manager suggested a possible change of times, but advised him to meet with his Moslem general practitioner to have the advice both medically and culturally confirmed.

Integrated or segregated services

The assumptions behind the idea of segregating service provision along lines of racial and cultural divides are that black people will have an assurance that their specific needs will be met, but also that the solution to eradicating the notion of racist practices will be transferred more to 'black' workers. This clearly fails to address the fundamental issues of the individual white practitioner's innate racist influences, which need resolution for the benefit of the practitioner and not just ethnic group service users. It also fails to address broader issues of institutional racism, which presumably would continue in all other aspects of a black person's interface with services and society. It also ignores the idea of choice for the small minority of people who are suspicious of the practitioners from their own ethnic group and may in fact choose a white professional.

Choice for the individual user can best be maximized through a primary focus on integrating services, whilst supporting the need for some segregated projects, e.g. the Fannon Project in Brixton, South London. The white service provider needs to be aware of how to access a range of culturally sensitive resources, whether they stand as integrated or segregated services.

GENDER

The statistics of psychiatric literature unanimously point to women using more services than men, with higher percentages of psychiatric diagnoses, higher percentage use of inpatient beds and outpatient clinics. Geller and Munetz (1988) propose a number of possible reasons for these findings, namely, that women accept mental illness in themselves more than men do, the sick role is more compatible than for men and the need to seek help is more accepted by women than men.

Bachrach and Nadelson (1988) suggest that the effects of chronic mental illness manifest themselves very differently for women and for men, with the implications that gender differences should inform and shape all aspects of clinical management. Yet the conclusions of Nicolson (1993) suggest that much clinical research and practice assumes a gender-free basis, which by default happens to conform more to a male model of practice. The recognition of gender differences appears to be a recent development in psychology, whereas previously women were simply seen as 'different from men' rather than uniquely equal (Nicolson and Ussher, 1992).

Inequality and injustice

The language of researchers and clinicians in relation to women and mental health tends to pin the cause very much on women's personality, ways of thinking, genetics, biochemistry and biology with little, if any, reference to the effects of social and sexual inequality through abuse, powerlessness, poverty, conflict and violence (Ussher, 1991). There is an equal tendency amongst practitioners to attribute blame through the typical labels of 'manipulation', 'overprotectiveness', 'weakness' and 'over-dependency' (Williams, 1993). This stereotyping of women with mental health problems has the effect of denying access to services that may meet unique needs, such as early pelvic examinations (Handel, 1988), and of making women feel punished by the services that they are in need of.

Sexual inequality is seen as a major cause of the despair, distress and confusion that have been labelled as women's mental illness. Williams (1993) also reports several studies to indicate that violence, sexual assault and abuse are root causes of what is diagnosed as mental illness for many women. The violence and abuse can be generalized to men, but it is also identified as occurring within the mental health services as well as outside, perpetrated not just by fellow patients but also by individual practitioners (Crossmaker, 1991).

Despite the growing evidence of causes rooted in social injustice, mental health practitioners are still trained and guided to focus on theories that uphold the identification of 'fault' in individuals, their bio-chemistry or their families (Williams, 1993). As with the case of racism, sexism clearly ignores the real and perceived effects of oppression and blame on the individual woman service user.

Gender differences

It is vitally important that service research and clinical practice continue to develop an understanding of the differences between men and women, so that a woman engaging in a working relationship may have confidence that her unique life experiences and needs will be addressed by service planning and delivery. Nicolson (1993) acknowledges that differences have both biological and social origins but the emphasis should be on social expectations framing the biological experience. It is also noted that:

> The differential value placed on particular achievements, e.g. parenthood, employment and promotion, appear to be weighted according to gender, and health professionals need to be aware that these are social constructions rather than 'intrinsic' qualities.
>
> (*Nicolson, 1993, p. 185*)

In terms of studies relating to chronic schizophrenia, Seeman (1988) notes gender differences in both onset age and response to neuroleptic medications. Bennett *et al.* (1988) studied institutional populations and observed women to be generally more interactive, demanding more time and attention. Men, on the other hand, were observed to be generally less verbally interactive but more physically threatening. They concluded that these significant differences should inform building design and service planning.

Role expectations

Psychological studies inform us that labelling through gender begins with parental expectations even before birth (Nicolson, 1993). Despite a recent relaxation of the sex role expectations, Johnstone (1989, p. 128) suggests a number of contrasts that still form the rule rather than the exception:

- Women are powerful in the family, men are powerful in the outside world.
- Men are allowed to be angry, women are allowed to be vulnerable.
- Women are permitted to be emotional, while men pride themselves on being rational.
- Men have power, women have relationships.
- Women are encouraged to care, men are expected to compete.

Despite the so-called advent of the 'new man', the above contrasts give some guidelines as to the historical culture that a potential female service user brings to the working relationship. The process of engagement and assessment should not lose sight of the likelihood that the woman has had to live with expectations that she should give more than she receives in relationships. She may frequently feel defined more in relation to others than in her own individual right, e.g. wife of ... or mother of ... Even where women come to the service with a previous or current history of employment, it is much more often in roles that entail giving and caring, for relatively lower remuneration.

Many women become conditioned to see their main role as carers and providers within the family unit, with lesser time for their own needs or a life outside of the family. Johnstone (1989) reminds us that this series of events is not so simply explained by the view of male domination, but it is also contributed to through the generations of mother–daughter relationships passing on the role model and expectations.

Whilst such role performance is not to be seen as intrinsically damaging in itself, we should be aware that problems begin to arise when the role is an enforced one, with little alternative choice and at the expense of the woman's own needs as a person. Personal resentment and crippling loss can be the consequences when the role is lost, as the children grow up and leave home. Some women blame themselves for many of their children's subsequent difficulties. Furthermore, Davis (1993) reminds us that as many women grow older and lose their primary roles, they are often left with little alternative identity and become increasingly devalued. It is important to remember all the while that such consequences, if they do arise, have stemmed from women simply doing what society has expected of them.

The psychiatric services frequently reinforce these role expectations. Women users are often seen to be treated successfully if they demonstrate a return to coping with domestic-based treatment programmes. A woman is then expected to return to the environmental situation that may have caused the initial distress. Any rebelling against expectations is frequently medicalized as 'aggressive' or 'non-compliant' behaviour and the sick role is reinforced.

Johnstone (1989) suggests that professionals frequently bring no greater understanding of the social implications of role expectations; in a number of studies, not even female professionals bring any guarantee of understanding how a woman's emotional distress may relate to the wider complex issues of women's roles. Davis (1993) suggests that psychiatry ultimately measures good mental health against masculine behaviours but if any woman displays these behaviours, it is regarded as abnormal, necessitating persuasive powers to adjust to a more feminine role. This adjustment is tagged as normal, but not necessarily as healthy on the objective research measures. In these ways, the medical approaches reinforce the stereotypes.

Practical service needs

Johnstone (1989) highlights the traditional focus on medical treatments for the woman who comes in to the psychiatric system:

> A vast pool of female distress is concealed by tranquillizers such as Valium. Women are prescribed these drugs far more often than men (the ratio has been estimated at about two to one), and this serves to obscure the underlying issues which are nearly always women's role problems.
>
> *(Johnstone, 1989, p. 119)*

As a result of the emphasis on using medication women are seen as the victims of inadequate service planning and are frequently lost in the community to otherwise much needed services (Bachrach and Nadelson, 1988).

Services that women consistently say that they want are a choice of women-only space, women workers, adequate childcare during periods of distress and opportunities to explore the underlying causes of distress (Davis, 1993). Added to this would be the need for all psychiatric staff to receive adequate training in gender issues.

Staff awareness

In relation to many of the issues outlined earlier in this chapter, Johnstone (1989) suggests that most psychiatric staff have little experience of what are predominantly women's problems, such as eating disorders and the emphasis on body image, childbirth, postnatal depression, abortion or miscarriage, or the victims of rape or a violent spouse, child sexual and physical abuse. Therefore, staff tend to unwittingly reinforce the predominant views expressed in society through having no higher degree of critical awareness of women's roles and unique experiences.

Not all women will present to the working relationship a catalogue of threats and abuses, but all are conditioned to role expectations to varying degrees and much of their more traumatic experience may remain firmly repressed until a uniquely trusting relationship is experienced. Consequently, staff need to be aware that hitherto unearthed material could suddenly be presented in the relationship.

Counselling approaches

The whole range of counselling skills discussed in Chapter 4 will be valid in the practical implementation of the working relationship with female service users. Davis (1993) suggests that counselling can play a major role in reducing the current widespread practice of prescribing medications, though it is still a relatively unconsidered option. The significance would be its emphasis on helping women to target issues of role expectations, particularly in helping to express feelings and validate their thoughts about themselves in relation to their significant others (Bennett *et al.*, 1988).

Counselling interventions present an alternative method whereby women can express their own needs and explore their own personal identity, free of the more traditional ties associated with gender roles. Johnstone (1989) suggests that up to now the sick role has been one of the few ways in which women could find some care and attention for themselves. She suggests that women need the encouragement to express the anger that many of them frequently suppress. Only an expression of true anger and frustration may open up paths for real change. The medical approaches to diagnosis and treatment have hitherto pinned fault to the individual woman and stifled any opportunity for change.

Unique physical needs

Bachrach and Nadelson (1988) suggest that one of the few successfully developed areas of support for chronically mentally ill women is that of family planning services. Important needs include counselling around sexuality, sex education, contraceptive services and advice, as well as education around legal and ethical issues of informed consent. Whilst all these issues are equally valid for men, it is women who frequently assume greater responsibility and become the victims of male irresponsibility.

Other gynaecological and physical needs are sadly not given the same level of attention. The reasons tend to focus around the chronically mentally ill frequently being viewed as 'genderless' (Bachrach and Nadelson, 1988) or else fear of skills erosion or malpractice suits against psychiatrists (Handel, 1988). Particular attention is drawn to the medical procedures of pelvic examinations, which though they are of vital importance to the healthcare of all women, are frequently 'deferred' by psychiatric staff. Handel (1988) suggests that the reasons why these examinations should be an integral part of medical checks are:

* psychiatric populations have a high incidence of physical illness;
* systems of community treatment are not comprehensive;
* women perceive pelvic examinations to be an important part of their general medical care;
* pelvic examinations may be life-saving procedures through early detection of life-threatening conditions.

Conversely, the reasons why such examinations are 'deferred' for many mentally ill women are:

* the chronically mentally ill person is often viewed as 'genderless';
* the psychiatric diagnosis can result in physical problems being overlooked;
* a potentially reduced ability to specify pain and discomfort;
* a psychiatrist's belief that the pelvic examination procedure may interfere with a special therapeutic relationship;
* a fear of malpractice suits;
* inexperience in performing physical examinations.

Work roles

In association with the function of counselling to free women from the restrictions of gender role expectations, practical measures need to be in place to fill the potential vacuum of activity. Recently there has been an upholding of equality of access to work opportunities, though the reality has been one of predominantly gender-related work roles. In addition, women have been expected to maintain multiple roles of both domestic duties and predominantly part-time low paid jobs. To extend this equality both sides of the equation need to be addressed: open access to all employment and training opportunities irrespective of gender and the sharing and support of other responsibilities around childrearing and domestic duties. Women wishing to retain control of childcare should be equally valued and supported to do so, whether through valuing the importance of the responsibility without taking it for granted or through measures that enable better access to child-care facilities in or near to the workplace.

Case study 7.4: Gena (34 years old)

Experiencing a progressive history of child physical abuse, teenage drug and alcohol abuse, anorexia through abusing laxatives, suicidal and mutilating responses to severe depressive episodes, Gena has consistently refused offers of medication on prescription and made some engagements in supportive and analytical psychotherapeutic approaches with varying degrees of success or reversion to self-destructive behaviours.

Despite some brief success working as a typesetter and commencing nursery nurse training, the death of her mother some four years ago triggered a relapse into patterns of self-destructive behaviour in response to waves of depression. Gena has a young family and a very supportive husband, who has learned to share childcare and domestic responsibilities around an adjustment to part-time work. Despite their own coping mechanisms, they both feel distrustful of statutory services following the sudden removal of their children into Social Services care, necessitating a long battle to secure their return.

In response to the family's requests, the introduction of the case management approach aims to target:

- the building of confidence through basic typesetting skills, to open up future employment and/or training opportunities;
- to reinstate the previously more successful 'supportive' rather than 'analytical' therapeutic approach;
- to help Gena focus on the positive achievements (however small they may seem), in order to challenge the more overwhelming negative self-image;
- to support the denial of medication;
- to help Gena look at her own denial around the extent of her destructive eating patterns.

SUMMARY

Since psychiatry is practised in a social setting, it is inevitable that the racist and sexist images, myths and expectations that are embedded deep within society will enter into and influence psychiatric theory and practice. The sociopolitical aspects of race, culture and gender cannot be separated from the engagement and development of the individual working relationship.

Fernando (1988) proposes a form of sociocultural practice that involves establishing a rapport with individual service users, requiring the practitioner to think and feel through the cultural viewpoints of the individuals concerned, including a cultural 'self-awareness'. It requires a sensitivity to the conceptual frameworks and experiences of the service user. Psychiatric disorder, as well as psychiatry itself, should be seen in the context of social influences, rather than through a purely medicalized approach.

We should strive to avoid stereotypes and exercise caution about making any generalizations. Stereotyping essentially results in missing the uniqueness of the individual, with a consequence that much needed and desired services and outcomes could be denied. We may only avoid the pitfall of stereotyping if we clearly identify the sociocultural context within which the interaction is taking place. We must also acknowledge 'difference' and work with its potentials, rather than diminishing our own understanding by assuming that everyone starts on a 'level playing field'.

REFERENCES

Bachrach, L.L. and Nadelson, C.C. (eds) (1988) *Treating Chronically Mentally Ill Women*, American Psychiatric Press, Washington.

Bavington, J. and Majid, A. (1986) Psychiatric services for ethnic minority groups, in *Transcultural Psychiatry*, (ed. J. Cox), Croom Helm, London, pp. 87–106.

Bennett, M.B., Handel, M.H. and Pearsall, D.T. (1988) Behavioral differences between female and male hospitalized chronically mentally ill patients, in *Treating Chronically Mentally Ill Women*, (eds L.L. Bachrach and C.C. Nadelson), American Psychiatric Press, Washington, pp. 29–44.

Brand, J. and McGinley, E. (1986) Power and prejudice. *Maudsley and Bethlem Gazette*, **31**(4), 14–16.

Crossmaker, M. (1991) Behind locked doors – institutional sexual abuse. *Sexuality and Disability*, **9**(3) 201–19.

D'Ardenne, P. and Mahtani, A. (1989) *Transcultural Counselling in Action*, Sage, London.

Davis, S. (1993) *THRESHOLD: A Local Initiative for Women and Mental Health*, Spring Newsletter, South East Thames Psychiatric Rehabilitation Interest Group.

Dominelli, L. (1988) *Anti-Racist Social Work*, Macmillan, London.

Dominelli, L. (1989) An uncaring profession? An examination of racism in social work. *New Community*, **15**(3), 391–403.

Eleftheriadou, Z. (1994) *Transcultural Counselling*, Gateway, London.

Fernando, S. (1988) *Race and Culture in Psychiatry*, Croom Helm, London.

Geller, J.L. and Munetz, M.R. (1988) The iatrogenic creation of psychiatric chronicity in women, in *Treating Chronically Mentally Ill Women*, (eds L.L. Bachrach and C.C. Nadelson), American Psychiatric Press, Washington, pp. 141–78.

Gobodo, P. (1992) Psychotherapy and culture, *Critical Health*, **32**, 52–8.

Guy's and Lewisham NHS Trust (1992) *Draft Code of Practice on Racial Discrimination in the Provision of Services*, Guy's and Lewisham NHS Trust, London.

Handell, M.H. (1988) Referred pelvic examinations: a purposeful omission in the care of mentally ill women, in *Treating Chronically Mentally Ill Women*, (eds L.L. Bachrach and C.C. Nadelson), American Psychiatric Press, Washington, pp. 97–110.

Johnstone, L. (1989) *Users and Abusers of Psychiatry. A Critical Look at Traditional Psychiatric Practice*, Routledge, London.

Lorde, A. (1984) *Sister Outsider*, The Crossings Press, New York.

Nicolson, P. (1993) Gender issues in ageing, in *Counselling and Psychology for Health Professionals*, (eds R. Bayne and P. Nicolson), Chapman & Hall, London, pp. 181–96.

Nicolson, P. and Ussher, J.M. (1992) *The Psychology of Women's Health and Health Care*, Macmillan, London.

Reber, A. (1985) *Dictionary of Psychology*, Penguin, Harmondsworth.

Seeman, M.V. (1988) Schizophrenia in women and men, in *Treating Chronically Mentally Ill Women*, (eds L.L. Bachrach and C.C. Nadelson), American Psychiatric Press, Washington, pp. 19–28.

Shackman, J. (1985) *A Handbook on Working with, Employing and Training Interpreters*, National Extension College, Cambridge.

Sue, D.W. and Sue, D. (1990) *Counselling the Culturally Different: Theory and Practice*, 2nd edn, Wiley, New York.

Ussher, J. (1991) *Women's Madness: Misogyny or Mental Illness?* Harvester Wheatsheaf, London.

Williams, J. (1993) *Women and Mental Health: Into the 1990s.* Spring Newsletter, South East Thames Psychiatric Rehabilitation Interest Group.

FURTHER READING

Banks, G. (1971) The effects of race on one-to-one helping interviews. *Social Service Review*, **45**, 137–46.

Brent Community Health Council (1981) *Black People and the Health Service*, Russell Press, Nottingham.

Chaplin, J. (1988) *Feminist Counselling in Action*, Sage, London.

Christie, Y. and Blunden, R. (1991) *Is Race on Your Agenda? Improving Mental Health Services for People from Black and Minority Groups*, King's Fund Centre, London.

Cox, J. (ed.) (1986) *Transcultural Psychiatry*, Croom Helm, London.

Littlewood, R. and Lipsedge, M. (1982) *Aliens and Alienists: Ethnic Minorities and Psychiatry*, Penguin, Harmondsworth.

Ussher, J.M. and Nicolson, P. (eds) (1992) *Gender Issues in Clinical Psychology*, Routledge, London.

Supervisory relationships: client supervision | 8

The concept of supervision carries significantly different connotations depending on the context in which it is being used. In general terms, a supervisor is a person who holds a degree of responsibility to oversee and direct the activities of another. This relationship may, however, be viewed very differently, on both sides, depending on how the power differential is interpreted and exercised. In one respect power may be presented quite negatively, through a sense of control and restriction. This exercising of supervision may frequently be accompanied by the strict definition of boundaries and goals, clearly defined by one person, imposed on another, ultimately even enforced by the use of sanctions or threats. Conversely, the idea of super-Vision can portray a more positive notion of support and enablement, exercised through encouragement, shared ideas and a valuing of the contribution an individual can make towards the definition of objectives to be achieved.

In the context of developing working relationships with people experiencing severe long-term mental health difficulties, the term supervision has become more synonymous with clients described as exhibiting destructive, aggressive or socially unacceptable behaviours. Consequently, it tends to be associated more with a restrictive and retributional approach, corrective of apparently maladaptive behaviour patterns. Until very recently the treatment approaches largely reflected a mood of society that favoured a more institutional approach, which raises the question whether 'supervision' is ultimately for the benefit of the individual or for the so-called protection of the general public. Accordingly, most of the literature has tended to focus on the clinical legislative and institutional issues and much less so on the clinical community care issues (Craft and Craft, 1984; Bluglass *et al.*, 1990).

With this in mind, it is hardly surprising that the whole notion of client supervision has become associated with issues of violence and aggression, largely linked to the associated functions of the criminal justice system. Its place within the mental health system appears to be strongly related to the functions of the special hospitals and the regional and local provision of secure unit beds. Even some of the earlier discussions of community supervision focused solely on the needs of the conditionally discharged patient who had previously been incarcerated in the hospital system (Norris, 1984).

More recent serious and fatal events have focused attention on the fact that many people in need of close supervision exist in the community and the less restrictive parts of the mental health system than occur in the special hospital services (Ritchie *et al.*, 1994). The criminal justice system and the specialist forensic psychiatry services have been required to acknowledge these wider service implications (DoH/Home Office, 1992). Furthermore, the legislative impact on mental health services has targeted priorities onto the needs of a large group of people requiring degrees of service supervision (DoH, 1990; NHS Management Executive, 1994).

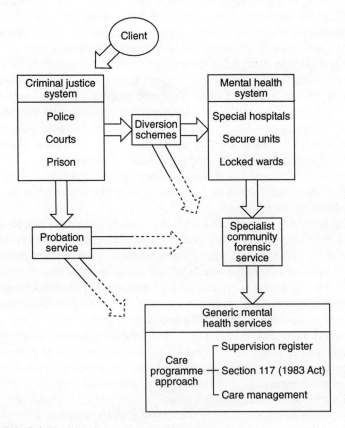

Figure 8.1 Criminal justice and mental health systems.

The previous narrow focus of attention onto 'mentally disordered offending' has now been opened up to include not just violence and aggression, but further serious risk-taking behaviours such as self-harm and severe self-neglect. The latter two categories of risk are generally considered to be more prevalent than the more commonly acknowledged factors of violence and threats of aggression.

The Department of Health (1993) highlights people with a history of aggression, risk-taking behaviours and offending as a particularly vulnerable client group. Inadequate supervision can only lead to an escalation of risk-taking behaviours with adverse consequences on their mental health. Whilst they present quite special problems for the process of assessment, Figure 8.1 illustrates the complexity of the systems in which they may become embroiled. Consequently, interagency collaboration presents a logistical problem, but one that of necessity needs to be successfully managed if we are to ensure continuity of care for the individual passing through the complex labyrinth of services and procedures. Crawford and Mee (1994) illustrate some of the difficulties in their reporting of how:

> Often an individual's first contact is with the criminal justice system (a prisoner); he/she may then move to a special hospital or a provider unit (a patient); and finally to a local authority (a client), where different aspects of care are provided. The difficulty for an individual can be that each of the organizations has a very different value system and method of working. ... (p. 26).

IMPLICATIONS FOR WORKING RELATIONSHIPS

The overriding factor to be appreciated by staff attempting to develop effective supervisory relationships with clients in the above system is the potential impact of environmental and legislative restrictions. The extreme form of environmental influence is compulsory detention in an institutional setting, with all the effects that long-term institutionalization may have on an individual. It is important to appreciate that staff also become contaminated by the influences of the institution, which engender systemized working practices. Goffman (1961) outlines a process of 'mortification' which can result in the institutionalized person losing their sense of personal identity, role and social relationship abilities. For staff it can become quite a difficult task to integrate the concepts of therapeutic intervention and necessary levels of security or to promote empowerment through personal choice when the primary service function is that of detention (Lloyd, 1995).

For clients experiencing lesser degrees of detention and security, there is still the impact of legislative restrictions which impact on the responsibilities and working practices expected of mental health practitioners. Even in the comparative freedom of the community there is still an expectation that services will be coordinated by an individual keyworker, who is charged with the task of maintaining contact and monitoring the progress of the client against stated goals. In itself, this may easily be interpreted as intrusive and restrictive; it certainly sits uneasily with the concepts of empowerment and choice and can lead to the practitioner role including 'social control', where the community becomes the client rather than the individual.

The use of terminology generally achieves the negative impact of a double stigma. Not only is a person labelled with all the connotations of long-term mental health problems, but they may also be frequently labelled 'mentally disordered offender', 'mentally abnormal offender' or 'forensic'. Declaration of such a history presents a major impediment to normal integration, where job opportunities are even more likely to be denied and prospective housing and support agencies are going to have their suspicions and fears raised about the potential for risk and danger.

An important impact on the process of relationship building will be an understanding of the client's own frame of reference, through appreciating the precipitants of their behaviours, their reappraisal of self-worth resulting from the impact of security and restriction (often heightening the risk of suicide or self-harm) and their need for specialized responsive community support from a system that has hitherto been very slow to develop in response to the special circumstances.

Furthermore, there is the whole question of how to undertake regular thorough risk assessment and to include adequate precautionary measures into the working practices. Such routine considerations must impact on the ability to develop effective working relationships. The expectation that practitioners may be able to accurately predict future risk-taking behaviours is a very difficult one; the most that can be expected is that a practitioner can access all relevant information on past behaviour patterns and incorporate this into the good practice of regular monitoring with the individual client.

POLICY GUIDANCE AND LEGISLATION

This history of security for mentally disordered offenders and other people deemed to be at risk is a relatively recent phenomenon. The evidence suggests a much greater weight of 'guidelines for practice' than actual legislation carrying the full legal backing of statutes of Parliament (Vaughan and Badger, 1995, Chapter 2).

Mental Health Act 1959

This introduced the need for special hospitals, to provide the required treatment under high security for people deemed to be mentally disordered and dangerous, violent or criminal in their behaviours. Responsibility for managing these services transferred from the Department of Health to a Special Hospitals Service Authority in 1989, though their specialized remit has ensured they remain marginalized from the mainstream provision of mental health services.

Home Office and Department of Health and Social Security (1975)

The Butler Report promoted the priority of forensic psychiatry services through provisions to establish regional secure units, with a target of 1000 beds nationally. The first RSU was not opened until 1980 and only 600 beds had been provided by the time of the Reed Report review in 1992.

Mental Health Act 1983

This is the main legislation governing the detention, treatment and supervised release of people with mental health problems, including mentally disordered offenders. Section 117 of the Act requires that health authorities and Social Services authorities have a duty to jointly assess the needs for support in the community of people who have been detained under Sections 3 or 37. It requires the nomination of a keyworker charged with the responsibility to coordinate regular reviews of the health and social care needs.

NHS and Community Care Act 1990

An attempt to integrate services to meet the needs of the most vulnerable people living in the community. Health and social care needs are to be more closely integrated, with local authorities becoming the lead agency for assessing individual need and arranging packages of care. The system of 'care management' was introduced to help prevent people with serious mental health problems slipping through the net of care. The care manager would act as a broker of services, with budgetary control to buy in services to meet individual needs of the client.

The care programme approach (Department of Health, 1990)

Health authorities and local authority Social Services departments are required to set up individually tailored packages of care for all people about to be discharged from inpatient units and for all new patients accepted by the specialist mental health services. The essential elements of an effective CPA are:

- a systematic assessment of health and social care needs (including accommodation);
- a care plan agreed between relevant professional staff, the patient and relevant carers;
- the allocation of a keyworker, to maintain regular contact, monitor delivery of the care plan and take action where it fails;
- regular review of the person's progress in relation to the agreed care plan.

The care programme approach is complementary to systems of care management. It differs in respect of the need for the keyworker to be involved in direct provision of care and the lack of direct budgetary control. The subsequent development of a care programme approach register is assumed to be the central feature of localized service administration and in some areas the care management information is being processed as a subregister of the CPA (Millington, 1994).

Department of Health and Home Office (1992)

The Reed Report focused a review of health and social care needs specifically on mentally disordered offenders and also represents an important watershed in the change of direction from predominantly secure inpatient facilities to needs in the community.

The main principles identified are:

- a regard to the quality of care and attention to individual needs;
- care and treatment should be provided through health and Social Services agencies rather than the criminal justice system;
- as far as possible care should be offered in the community rather than the institution, but with appropriate security observed;
- opportunities should access skills rehabilitation to maximize personal independence;
- people should be in, or as near as possible to, their own local area and/or family.

The fundamental issues addressed by the numerous recommendations are:

- the need for a positive approach to individual needs;
- a multidisciplinary/multiagency approach;
- an improved range of community services;
- an expansion of medium secure and 'outreach' services;
- contracting of healthcare from the NHS for prisoners;
- improved general and specialist forensic psychiatry training.

The Reed Report stresses the need for better coordination and effective use of current resources, but also a substantial need for new resources (Flood, 1993).

Supervision registers (NHS Management Executive, 1994)

In essence, the supervision register is a subset of the care programme approach. It is a requirement of all health authorities that they ensure the establishment and maintenance of a register that details information on people with a severe mental illness who are believed to be at a significant risk to themselves or others, whether through violence, self-harm or severe self-neglect. This guidance takes forward the policy of ensuring that those patients subject to the CPA who pose most risk receive adequate care, support and supervision in the community. Judgements of risk should be based on detailed evidence of past psychiatric and social history and current condition (including consultations with all health, Social Services and criminal justice agencies, as appropriate). Clearly identified warning signs should be recorded on the register documentation.

Criticisms of the guidance focus on the lack of new resources for its implementation (Holloway, 1994) and the potential infringement of liberties through the lack of any appeal process against the decision of inclusion (Vaughan and Badger, 1995). Tyrer and Kennedy (1995) prefer to highlight its potential benefits for targeting the people most at risk, seeing it more for its administrative and procedural functions. However, the guidance on targeting needy individuals has been open to wide local interpretations, possibly failing its intention to provide a unified national register (McCarthy et al., 1995).

With regard to the working relationship, it is the consultant psychiatrist, not the keyworker, who makes the final decision of inclusion on the register and informs the patient of this status. However, the keyworker, as party to the multidisciplinary discussions that inform the decision, is still subject to the influences that presentation of the information may have on subsequent working relationships:

- negative presentation: linked to the discussions around the potential for compulsory community treatment, with threats of removal to hospital if the person does not comply with the stated care plan;
- positive presentation: a method of targeting limited resources so that those most in need are ensured an agreed level of contact. Also a method of offering regular assessment for people deemed to be at severe risk.

The register itself is only a means of administrative documentation. The implementation of its practical intentions is awaited through a Mental Health Bill to Parliament, which will amend the Mental Health Act 1983.

The fears surrounding any changes to the legislation are the introduction of new powers of compulsory detention in certain circumstances of non-compliance with details for care and support. The tension in the debate arises between those advocating more powers of treatment and the civil liberties lobby. The difficulty for the individual service user and service practitioner is the question of how to build a relationship of trust in such a climate; a relationship that serves to promote a central principle of the care programme approach, that of treatment plans being arrived at by mutual negotiation rather than one-sided compulsion (Fulop, 1995).

Inclusion on the supervision register should ensure:

- a keyworker who is an experienced community mental health professional;
- an allocated social worker;
- registration with a general practitioner;
- a multidisciplinary assessment of health and social care needs;
- a care plan attending to individual risk and needs;
- regular multidisciplinary reviews;
- a forensic assessment within six months.

Particular attention will be drawn in the next sections to the implications of assessing and responding to risk, within the supervisory relationship.

RISK ASSESSMENT

The concepts of risk-taking behaviours and risk assessment have become fashionable for scrutiny in current mental health practice. This is partly in response to the recent media profile of a small number of 'extreme' incidents, highlighting the need for central government to declare its priorities for resource management. Consequently, public awareness and associated fears of the potential and real damages of psychiatric disturbance are heightened. The issues are ever present for service users and practitioners and of necessity should always be respected as an integral and continuing element of assessment practices.

Institutional settings of medium to high security, e.g. the special hospitals and secure units, have a built-in advantage regarding the assessment and responses to risks. Whilst the pressure cooker effect of high security institutional living may predispose to higher incidences of risk behaviours, the frequency of contact and well-rehearsed routines of intervention and containment enable a more continuous assessment and response to potential and actual situations (Lloyd, 1995).

The situation outside the institution presents a very different set of circumstances. Vaughan and Badger (1995) remind us that:

> By contrast, workers in the community are far more exposed to risk with considerably less support. Their clients are much more likely to be unknown quantities in terms of risk potential. Opportunities to get close to the client in order to pick up early signs of difficulties are often limited to brief contacts ... once or twice a week ... Furthermore, many are notoriously difficult to keep track of ... (p. 79).

People experiencing long-term mental health problems, particularly with a potential for risk-taking behaviours, are at a high risk around the point of discharge from inpatient units to the community. This is a time of increased ambivalence, as they are about to transfer from a situation of high interpersonal contact to one of potential isolation and infrequent contacts with others. The picture is also confused by the tension between the value of the working relationship and its potential to be restrictive on freedom and independence, even to the degree of social control where elements of supervision are linked as conditions of discharge (Vaughan and Badger, 1995).

One of the particular challenges presented to the relationship by the need for risk assessment is that of predicting future risk-taking behaviours. In light of the ambivalences and contradictions outlined above, the art of prediction becomes a particularly difficult business. In many walks of life the unpredictability of human nature is regarded as a virtue but not so when the potential for violence or self-harm is high. Whittington and Wykes (1994) report on several studies into the prediction of violence, but they suggest: ' ... The conclusion from these studies seems to be that a large number of assaults are not anticipated by staff, even though the staff may have been experienced and qualified in assessing people's behaviour' (p. 155).

Whilst the limitations of practice in this area are quite evident, we need to be clear as to what is best practice in the current level of knowledge. Certainly the need for supervising relationships with clients should incorporate elements of risk assessment and precautionary practices as an integral and continuous part of our work. We should, however, acknowledge the influence that these practices may have on the relationship, e.g. do they demonstrate to the client our perpetual state of fear about their behaviour or do they present an element of reassuring safe professional practice?

RISK OF AGGRESSION AND VIOLENCE

These are the elements of risk that excite most media attention, yet serious incidents are relatively rare and certainly less common than examples of self-harm and severe self-neglect. Whittington (1994) reports on 'the assaultive patient', based on studies of psychiatric hospital populations. The results suggest that only a minority of patients act aggressively and a very small proportion of this minority are repeatedly aggressive. However, the fact is that incidents do occur and the impact of psychiatric disturbance on human behaviour is comparatively unpredictable with potentially serious or fatal results, which indicates the importance of assessing and accommodating risks.

Aggression

This is commonly a behavioural expression of anger, though sometimes it may be an expression of attention seeking in the absence of anger. Aggression in itself may not always present a problem. It has a place in everyday living, as a means of providing a safety valve or keeping others at a distance. It may also be a method of forcing overdue decisions to be made or actions to be taken, through its way of increasing the tempo. As a specific instrument of behaviour it may be operated within certain controlling limits by the perpetrator; however, when normal controls on acceptable limits fail then violence occurs.

Violence

This is a more extreme and dramatic expression of feelings such as anger, fear or despair. In certain circumstances it may also be used as a more primitive response for redressing perceived or real imbalances of power in the interpersonal relationship. There is no clearly agreed definition of violence, because it covers such a wide range of potential situations and circumstances. Burns (1993) quotes an earlier Department of Health and Social Security definition:

> The application of force, severe threat or serious abuse ... (including) Severe verbal abuse or threat where this is judged likely to turn into actual violence; serious or persistent harassment (including racial or sexual harassment); threat with a weapon; major or minor injury; fatalities (p. 53).

Clearly the incidence of aggression or violence will affect the relationship by introducing degrees of caution into the recipient's behaviour. However, there is no evidence to support a persistent fear of imminent violence; as Whittington and Wykes (1994) remind us: ' ... violence rarely takes place "out of the blue", without some behavioural change immediately beforehand' (p. 168).

Factors in the risk assessment

The individual client

1. Ensure you have all available information on:
   - mental state and physical condition;
   - social functioning;
   - past history of behaviours;
   - defining situations or warning signs, e.g. drug and/or alcohol abuse, stopping medication, specific interpersonal triggers (high expressed emotion).
2. Access to all sources of information:
   - self-reports at interview;
   - observing discrepancies between client verbal report and practitioner observations;
   - team members, carers, friends, relatives, police, probation, other statutory and voluntary services.
3. Personality factors:
   - cultural/subcultural values related to violence;
   - parental attitudes and childrearing behaviours;
   - repeated exposure to aggression and/or violence;
   - failure to learn delaying gratification of wants;
   - failure to develop alternative strategies;
   - repeated impulsive behaviours;
   - inability to cope with stress or frustration.
4. Physical warning signs:
   - clenched fists;
   - pacing/walking briskly;
   - throwing objects;
   - exaggerated responses to annoyance;
   - pressured and/or louder speech;
   - rigid muscle tension;
   - verbal threats;
   - invading personal space/disinhibited behaviour.

Wykes (1994) reminds us that any significant change from the 'normal' for the individual should be taken seriously as a sign of things possible.

The individual worker

1. Uninformed about important information regarding the client or the environment.
2. Inexperienced or poorly trained for working with particular client groups or conducting risk assessments.

3. Working alone in difficult circumstances or feeling unsupported by the team or management structure.

The meeting environment

1. Physical layout:
   • home, ward, office, centre;
   • positioning of furniture;
   • clear exit routes;
   • extremes of temperature;
   • overcrowding.
2. Presence of potential weapons.
3. Indirect effects on emotional arousal:
   • long waiting times;
   • staff focus on own routine above client needs;
   • poor explanations of procedures.

The community

1. Housing estates with known reputations for risk.
2. Gangs of youths.
3. Timing of visits, day or night.
4. Poor street lighting or broken lifts.
5. Threats from dogs, owned or stray.
6. Threats from the client's carers, friends or neighbours.

There are many factors that constitute a thorough risk assessment but not all of these would be immediately noticeable in the direct context of the working relationship. In many aspects, risk assessment is about the good working practice of advanced preparation and the laying down of foundations for procedures or actions to be implemented rapidly when necessary. Too much overt security and outward concern or fear give off the wrong type of messages, that subsequently fuel and intensify risk behaviours rather than achieving the intention of reducing risk.

Precautions for reducing risk

1. Satisfactory procedures:
   • for information gathering;
   • for using team discussions to focus on risk assessment;
   • for regular reviews in supervision or clinical meetings;
   • for joint working in situations of expected risk;
   • for developing team responsibility for assessing risks;

- for office organization, e.g. diaries of staff whereabouts and expected times of return;
- for assessing locations;
- for establishing escape routes and access to emergency services, if needed.

2. Clear plans:
   - based on information from all sources;
   - being clear about time and purpose of each visit;
   - use of contracts and boundaries, where relevant;
   - good communication between services.
3. Common sense:
   - by keeping safety and precautions on your personal agenda;
   - by asking for help;
   - through clarity of purpose;
   - by never allowing a good relationship to reduce caution and induce complacency.

The impact on the relationship will be more recognizable through the precautions enacted in the direct contact, most specifically:

- the practitioner's approach through the use of counselling skills (see Chapter 4), e.g. active listening, and allowing time for anger to be expressed and dissipated;
- open and non-confrontational questioning;
- non-judgemental responses;
- role model calmer non-verbal communications, but without encroaching on the need for wider personal space at times of anger;
- assessing the directedness of verbal threats of aggression;
- leaving the scene if the threats are immediate and directed towards you. Do not retaliate, physically or verbally.

The value of accurate information about past behaviours and warning signs lies in its regular use as prompts to questioning about current mental state and intended actions. Such information should be used for educational purposes, where possible, to help the individual service user understand their own early warning signs more clearly. A trusting relationship may be developed and enhanced by positive sharing of the monitoring task; this may also help the client to experience a more empowering relationship.

Case study 8.1 Tony (37 years old)

Experiencing a psychiatric history diagnosed with a paranoid psychotic illness since the early 1990s. The picture is complicated by long-standing alcohol abuse and a criminal record of minor offences over a 20-year period. Tony experienced an escalation of the seriousness of his offending behaviour in 1991 that was clearly linked to the development of psychiatric problems. He was initially charged with assault and criminal damage; he developed a 'hit-list' of ten people and was finally arrested for assault causing grievous bodily harm with a knife on the person heading his list. A period of imprisonment and psychiatric assessment lead on to formal detention in hospital on a section of the Mental Health Act 1983 and subsequent assessment for placement on the Supervision Register.

Risk precautions
- Initial community contacts were made in an outpatient clinic and home visits were jointly organized by two members of staff from the community team or one person in conjunction with the allocated social worker.
- Regular questioning of Tony about his 'paranoid' feelings, any re-development of a 'hit-list' and potential for accidentally meeting his previous victim in the street.
- Subsequent development of a trusting relationship has enabled staff to visit Tony alone.
- Close monitoring of medication compliance with GP practice staff.
- Regular discussion with Tony of potential early warning signs of relapse into a psychotic condition.

Positive developments
- Tony is able to slowly negotiate reductions of his antipsychotic medication.
- Tony has engaged in a few counselling sessions to discuss his insight into the development of previous dangerously unfortunate circumstances.
- Placement on a Supervision Register is seen as a way of ensuring continuity of services Tony finds helpful.
- Plans to access work rehabilitation training, towards the longer term goal of employment.
- Tony enjoys a number of established friendships that offer him invaluable support.

Management after an incident

Not all incidents of violence are avoided or indeed avoidable. In the unfortunate aftermath of an incident it is important that all involved people are offered the fullest support. For the client it can be a learning experience to talk through with the involved member of staff or more probably another person. Retrospective insight into the effect of a mental health problem on a person's behaviour can bring intense feelings of guilt, shame or remorse, which require sensitive handling.

The involved member of staff should talk through the incident with their supervisor, manager and/or team as appropriate to the situation. Apart from the need for support, it can also be an opportunity for the individual and the service as a whole to assess working practices. Wykes (1994) reminds us that the worker may occasionally be in the complicated situation of returning to the role of carer in a relationship with their assailant. However, the nature of the incident and impact on those involved may clearly dictate that any previous working relationship is damaged beyond repair, requiring a reallocation of work.

Aggression and violence towards clients

The whole of this discussion has so far assumed the client to be the assailant and the worker to be the victim. Despite the foundations of professional training, thorough staff induction and work experience and the development of supportive supervisory structures, human nature being the unpredictable factor that it is, some clients still end up as the victims of acts of worker aggression or violence. We all have a duty to assess, report and protect individual clients from the malpractices of irresponsible workers. The client also has a right to the same emotional and practical support that would be offered to an aggrieved worker. They also have a right to expect that the necessary and relevant disciplinary and/or criminal actions may be taken against the offending worker, including dismissal from employment if appropriate.

RISK OF SUICIDE AND SELF-HARM

People experiencing severe long-term mental health problems generally, and more specifically the group of people requiring closer supervisory relationships, are known to exhibit higher than average risks of suicide and self-harm. Consequently, the *Health of the Nation* targets (DoH, 1993) specify a reduction of suicide rates for the severely mentally ill by at least 33% by the year 2000. Furthermore, the spectacularly violent methods sometimes adopted by people in the depths of despair tend to draw wider media and public attention, somehow satisfying the 'newsworthiness of the gruesome detail'.

Vaughan (1985) identifes two subgroups of suicidal response:

1. Overwhelmed by an individual disaster but lacking the necessary support or personal coping mechanisms, despite an otherwise stable personal background.
2. Prolonged psychological instability and social disruption, perhaps characterized by several attempts at suicidal behaviour and/or antisocial behaviours.

Most people in this client group would tend to fall into the second category and can present serious challenges to the relationship with a service practitioner, primarily because of the perpetual threat of self-destructive behaviours in the light of deep despair and low self-esteem. However, risk assessment in this category is not focused entirely on suicide potential; we are concerned with four categories of behaviour:

1. suicidal behaviour with planned intent;
2. suicidal behaviour as a call for help;
3. cutting and mutilation as a call for help or attention;
4. self-abusing and addictive behaviours.

Factors in the assessment of risk

1. Statistical inferences:
   - more women attempt, more men succeed;
   - single, separated, divorced and widowed people are more likely to attempt suicide than married people;
   - age-related components point to an increased incidence in the over-50s;
   - cultural components, e.g. Asian women and white unemployed males in late teens and early 20s.
2. Alcohol and drug abuse.
3. At the time of hospital discharge and community resettlement.
4. Previous history of suicide attempts (including a family history).
5. Definite statements of planned intent.
6. Degree of irreversibility of plans and an absence of other people in close proximity (in stated plan).
7. A catalogue of recent negative life events.
8. Rejection of available support systems at a time of increased vulnerability and/or despair.

Communication and risk

The most obvious warning sign is a direct statement of planned intent; there is no truth in the myth that people who talk about suicide do not enact it. The DoH (1994) states that two-thirds of people who commit suicide have mentioned their intentions to other people, including GPs and specialist mental health professionals. Within the working relationship staff need to develop a sensitivity to subtle cries for help or statements of planned intent. It is important not to allow your anxieties about the serious content of the discussion to cloud listening skills. Tactful direct enquiries about intentions do not make them more likely to happen. On the contrary, the risk may be reduced by the implicit communication of understanding and concern that arises from direct discussion of plans and possible outcomes. Vaughan and Badger (1995) discuss this valuable intervention; through sharing the assessment of risk with the client, you may help them to evaluate the degree of control they can exercise over their potentially destructive actions.

However, for some people (in a very small minority), no amount of sharing risk assessment or interventions can take away the intensity of feeling. Suicide may be the only solution and as devastating as it will always be, the practitioner needs to be aware of their limits to help within the relationship.

Case study 8.2: Gena (34 years old)

Also detailed in Case Study 7.4, Gena has a long history of destructive behaviours including:

- alcohol and drug abuse;
- suicide attempts;
- self-mutilating through cutting her arms;
- abusing laxatives and Epsom salts;
- family and marital relationship difficulties.

Suicide plan
Gena initially raised a question with her workers about the likelihood of successfully killing herself, if she were to drop a piece of electrical equipment into the bath with her. The initial questioning developed into checking out the potential for her young children to be electrocuted by coming back to the home after she had killed herself; and whether such an action may cause a fire that would endanger others. At one point she planned to drink sufficient alcohol to numb the pain of the following actions and planned to leave the key in the locked front door to stop her family suddenly gaining entry to the home, thus putting themselves at risk.

Assessment of risk
Gena's clear development of a plan, with her need to check out the different eventualities in order that she may further refine her intentions, is an example of a high risk. She suggests that discussing the plan in detail with her workers does help to relieve some of the intense pain and gives her the means to acknowledge the control she has over her own actions. Gena has attempted suicide within hospital before, so removing her from home would not necessarily achieve the aim of saving her life. On the contrary, her main reasons for living are at home, particularly her children's need for her.

The other focus of intervention is to explore the escape valve of going out from home, at an early stage of despair, leading to the initiation of the planned actions. Gena has a list of local destinations she could walk to (written in large letters), pinned up on the kitchen wall (the room where she most frequently sits and ruminates on her suicidal ideas).

RISK OF SEVERE SELF-NEGLECT

For the general client group of people experiencing severe long-term mental health problems, this category of risk is probably of the most frequent incidence, yet attracts the lowest priority. The reason for this is that incidences of aggression or self-harm are more immediate in their impact than the more protracted process of self-neglect. At most, it may be attributed to an acclimatization, or even a level of acceptance, that some people with severe mental health problems live in conditions of squalor and neglect.

To be considered a risk, self-neglect must be severe enough to lead to:
1. the development of a serious 'physical illness' or disability;
2. the relapse into a serious 'mental state' that would endanger general health and well-being;
3. the development of a serious 'environmental health' problem that may endanger the client, carers or other visitors.

Factors in the assessment of risk

1. A previous history of repeated severe self-neglect, including environmental health problems through deteriorating condition of the accommodation (possibly necessitating the use of council environmental health services for cleaning or clearance).
2. A progressively deteriorating physical condition, denied by the client.
3. Repeated non-compliance with medical treatment and/or support.
4. A progressive denial and neglect of personal hygiene and general daily living skills.
5. The hoarding of rubbish or persistent neglect of rotting food.
6. A denial of danger from malfunctioning appliances, e.g. cooker or fire.
7. The disconnection of essential services, e.g. water, gas, electricity.
8. Leaving home with doors unlocked or open.

N.B. A combination of a number of factors is needed in order to attribute a high level of risk.

Relationship implications

The levels of neglect involved here will generally imply a denial of the need for, or even a rejection of, support. It may require the practitioner to revise their expectations of a working relationship to a lower level of negotiating specific functions or activities that may support 'survival' rather than 'personal growth' for the client. Attempts to inform and educate about the dangers or of the minimum standards that could invoke legal actions may help the client to focus on the worst consequences of neglect.

Otherwise, it becomes an exercise of monitoring to the point of formal detention under the Mental Health Act 1983 or the instigating of actions by the Environmental Health department of the local council. The latter options scarcely indicate a satisfactory development of a relationship, but may be necessary actions in the interests of a person's safety.

Case study 8.3: Mary (58 years old)

Further details are discussed in Case Study 5.6. Mary effectively neglects her personal hygiene and appearance, made worse by the effects of a prolapsed bowel staining her clothing and furniture and hormonal problems causing the growth of facial hair. Mary has persistently refused offers of help to attend to her appearance and the cleanliness of her home, frequently denying that there is any problem. Her cooker has been previously disconnected because of the potential dangers of use with her extrapyramidal tremors in both hands. Meals-on-wheels have been provided to support her diet.

Work with Mary has partly focused on what she needs to do to avoid people seeking legal powers to override her decisions to refuse help. As a result she does accept:

- all prescribed medications;
- the need for daily meals-on-wheels;
- the need to remove at least the remnants of food before it presents environmental health hazards;
- the need to accept help and advice with claiming benefits and paying necessary bills.

FURTHER CONSIDERATIONS FOR GOOD PRACTICE

Good practice must begin with better quality and more accessible staff training in the skills of working with client groups who require greater levels of 'supervision'. In addition to the areas already discussed around risk assessment, detention and assessment of early warning signs, staff also need to develop their own attitudes and awareness of realistic expectations in line with degrees of security or supervision. However liberal an approach we may wish to adopt, there is still the imposition of legal restrictions that occasionally governs the availability of possible options.

Diversion schemes

Initiated through the Home Office (1990), this was seen as a method of diverting those people from the criminal justice system who would better be served by receiving appropriate treatment and support from the statutory health and Social Services authorities. However, a report by Jones (1992) criticized the schemes as generally failing to meet the needs of mentally vulnerable people processed by the criminal justice system, because the limited resources of the statutory services were already inundated with competing demands from different user groups. The report initiated a pilot project, the 'Revolving Doors Agency', to provide a multidisciplinary diversion and community care service that would access and ensure continuity of needed service provisions for mentally disordered offenders, for whom diversion into mainstream community services appeared to be a reasonable option.

The remit of this agency to provide the link between the criminal justice system and the mainstream mental health system highlights the vitally important need for strengthening the network of support that may develop around any particular individual. Despite the undesirability of accommodating a mentally disordered offender in the criminal justice system, there is little to be gained from diversionary action if all that happens is a person floundering in the community and resorting to offending behaviours again. Consequently, there needs to be a comprehensive range of general and specialist community services, including a range of advocacy services, that can provide effectively for the complex and challenging needs of such people.

Case management approaches

The principles and practice of ideas from case management have been detailed throughout this text, but most specifically in Chapters 3 and 5. Table 8.1 outlines contrasting styles of providing community services to people subject to 'supervisory' relationships. These styles are not established as mutually exclusive extremes but need further exploring in each local service context, to see how they may be merged to present an effective and empowering experience for people more used to the influence of restrictive measures controlling them.

Table 8.1 Styles of community treatment

Case management	Community supervision
Engagement	Legislation
Promotional	Restrictive
Strengths	Problems
Choices	Compulsion
Empowering	Disempowering

The strengths model could be beneficially employed, within legal constraints and expectations, to help individual service users explore their own desires and future plans. Looking more specifically at what needs to be achieved to avoid a return to the criminal justice system concentrates the focus of attention away from the more immediate impact of current security and restrictions. This approach may also mesh quite satisfactorily with work on early warning signs of relapse and the precipitants of risk-taking behaviours.

Once again we are concerned to develop relationships with people who are not in contact with services necessarily by personal choice and in this case may be severely restricted against their will. The positive promotion of assertive outreach may be an essential aspect of developing a relationship, taking precedence over the more usual request to attend appointments supported by the persuasive back-up of recall under legal powers for non-attendance.

Interpersonal skills

The therapeutic and supportive relationship skills, discussed in Chapters 4 and 5 respectively, are of equal value in the context of working within supervisory relationships.

Listening, attending, empathy and genuine concern are just as vital for establishing the trust necessary for an effective working relationship with someone under supervision for risk-taking behaviours. Indeed, the need to possibly be more intrusive into regular monitoring of mental state and precipitants of risk-taking behaviours may be presented in a more user-friendly manner if staff adopt an attitude that these skills can be usefully applied. True equality in the relationship may be difficult to achieve fully, in view of certain restrictive requirements, but it should still be aimed for by the practitioner as much as possible. It is also arguable whether true empathic understanding can be achieved, as the practitioner would rarely have the experience of the user, but we should still aim for good quality empathy through an openness to the experiences of the client.

Practical life skills

Garner (1995) suggests:

> For those who have had a prolonged period of illness and/or hospital care, there must be a consistent level of stimulation and pressure in order to motivate them towards change. The patient must understand how the world has changed while he has been ill and how this illness has changed him ....

She advocates the importance of a flexible programme of work preparation and skills to help people achieve one of their more important priorities on return to the community, that of employment or meaningful activity.

The double stigma of mental illness and offending or risk-taking behaviour presents considerable barriers to full reintegration into the community. The full skills of a competent multidisciplinary team should be employed to address the range of issues from housing, employment and money to emotional support, coping mechanisms, daily living skills and use of leisure time. However, it is the individual keyworker 'supervisory' relationship that provides the focal point for the motivation to access the wider range of service opportunities.

SUMMARY

Until recently the predominant focus of service provision for people exhibiting mentally disordered and risk-taking behaviours was the institutional forensic psychiatric services (Lloyd, 1995). The Reed Report (DoH/Home Office, 1992) gave a renewed impetus for the direction of new resources into community forensic support. Up to this point the community focus was more concerned with the relationship between the Probation Service and specialist outreach forensic assessments. The danger is one of strengthening the interface between specialized institutional and community forensic services, with little or no further resources for the generic mental health teams who still have responsibility for a 'supervision register' client group who continue to cause significant public concern.

The influences of legislative restrictions can impact significantly on the development of a supervisory relationship. The question arises whether the supervisory process is primarily to promote individual freedom or public safety; who is the client, the individual or the community (Vaughan and Badger, 1995)?

The work requires a cooperative team approach taking into account the specific needs of the individual, the family and extended network of care, the psychosocial and environmental issues. The environment is influenced by levels of security, control and fears of risk-taking behaviour, which may sometimes take precedence over the promotion of treatment and support. Service coordination needs to take account of many providers across both the criminal justice and mainstream mental health systems (Lloyd, 1995).

An effective risk assessment will identify the relevant factors involved in past behaviour, indicate the circumstances which may act as future precipitants of risk and estimate the likelihood of these recurring. The multidisciplinary team and informal carers should be aware of an assessment and ensure prompt reappraisal if the factors indicate an increased risk.

It is important to note that the majority of people are not in contact with services by choice. This suggests that the development of effective supervisory relationships calls on a range of therapeutic and supportive skills and may benefit from an assertive outreach approach, adopting principles of case management, with careful coordination of the full network of care providers.

REFERENCES

Bluglass, R., Bowden, P. and Walker, B. (eds) (1990) *Principles and Practice of Forensic Psychiatry*, Churchill Livingstone, Edinburgh.

Burns, J. (1993) Working with potential violence, in *Counselling and Psychology for Health Professionals*, (eds R. Bayne and P. Nicolson), Chapman & Hall, London, pp. 51–64.

Craft. M. and Craft, A. (1984) *Mentally Abnormal Offenders*, Baillière Tindall, London.

Crawford, M. and Mee, J. (1994) The role of occupational therapy in the rehabilitation of the mentally disordered offender. Report of College of Occupational Therapy study day. *British Journal of Occupational Therapy*, **57**(1), 26–8.

Department of Health (1990) *The Care Programme Approach for People with a Mental Illness Referred to the Specialist Psychiatric Services*. HC(90)23, LASSL(90)11, Department of Health, London.

Department of Health/Home Office (1992) *Review of Health and Social Services for Mentally Disordered Offenders: Final Summary Report*. CM 2088, HMSO, London.

Department of Health (1993) *The Health of the Nation. Key Area Handbook: Mental Illness*, HMSO, London.

Department of Health (1994) *Draft Guidance: Discharge of Mentally Disordered People and their Continuing Care in the Community*, Department of Health, London.

Flood, B. (1993) Implications for occupational therapy services following the Reed Report. *British Journal of Occupational Therapy*, **56**(8), 293–4.

Fulop, N. (1995) Mental health: cash in the community. *The Guardian*, Society supplement (8.3.95).

Garner, R. (1995) Prevocational training within a secure environment: a programme designed to enable the forensic patient to prepare for mainstream opportunities. *British Journal of Occupational Therapy*, **58**(1), 2–6.

Goffman, E. (1961) Asylums, Doubleday, New York.

Holloway, F. (1994) Supervision registers: recent government policy and legislation. *Psychiatric Bulletin*, **18**, 593–6.

Home Office (1990) *Provision for Mentally Disordered Offenders*. Home Office Circular No. 66/90, London.

Home Office and Department of Health and Social Security (1975) *Report of the Committee on Mentally Abnormal Offenders*. Cmnd 6244, HMSO, London.

Jones, H. (1992) *Revolving Doors: Report of the Telethon Inquiry into the Relationship Between Mental Health, Homelessness and the Criminal Justice System*, NACRO, London.

Lloyd, C. (1995) *Forensic Psychiatry for Health Professionals*, Chapman & Hall, London.

McCarthy, A., Roy, D., Holloway, F. *et al.* (1995) Supervision registers and the care programme approach: a practical solution. *Psychiatric Bulletin*, **19**, 195–9.

Millington, C. (1994) The development of the care programme approach in North Derbyshire. *Occupational Therapy News*, **2**(3), 13.

NHS and Community Care Act (1990) HMSO, London.

NHS Management Executive (1994) *Introduction of Supervision Registers for Mentally Ill People from 1st April, 1994*. Health Service Guidelines HSG(94)5, London.

Norris, M. (1984) *Integration of Special Hospital Patients into the Community*, Gower, Aldershot.

Ritchie, J.H., Dick, D. and Lingham, R. (1994) *The Report of the Inquiry into the Care and Treatment of Christopher Clunis*. Presented to the Chairmen of North East Thames and South East Thames Regional Health Authorities, HMSO, London.

Tyrer, P. and Kennedy, P. (1995) Supervision registers: a necessary component of good psychiatric practice. *Psychiatric Bulletin*, **19**, 193–4.

Vaughan, P.J. (1985) Suicide Prevention, Pepar Publications, Birmingham.

Vaughan, P.J. and Badger, D. (1995) *Working with the Mentally Disordered Offender in the Community*, Chapman & Hall, London.

Whittington, R. (1994) Violence in psychiatric hospitals, in *Violence and Health Care Professionals*, (ed. T.Wykes), Chapman & Hall, London, pp. 23–43.

Whittington, R. and Wykes, T. (1994) The prediction of violence in a health care setting, in *Violence and Health Care Professionals,* (ed. T. Wykes), Chapman & Hall, London, pp. 155–73.

Wykes, T. (ed.) (1994) *Violence and Health Care Professionals*, Chapman & Hall, London.

FURTHER READING

Carson, D. (ed.) (1990) *Risk-taking in mental disorder: Analyses, Policies and Practical Strategies*, SLE Publications, Chichester.

Gardner, R. (1995) Prevocational training within a secure environment: a programme designed to enable the forensic patient to prepare for mainstream opportunities. *British Journal of Occupational Therapy*, **58**(1), 2–6.

Herbst, K.R. and Gunn, J. (eds) (1991) *The Mentally Disordered Offender*, Butterworth-Heinemann, Oxford.

Lloyd, C. (1995) Trends in forensic psychiatry. *British Journal of Occupational Therapy*, **58**(5), 209–13.

Yates, J.F. (ed.) (1992) *Risk-taking Behaviour*, Wiley, Chichester.

Supervisory relationships: staff supervision

The concept of supervision applied to service users, whatever the approach that is adopted, will still have to take account of the need for some level of restriction, either imposed through legal requirements or the expedience of personal safety for self or others. Initially, staff supervision may often be greeted with scepticism, being seen as a management tactic for checking on people, searching out and penalizing poor performance or applying pressure to increase productivity. However, in general, it is intended as a positive function of the organization, for supporting and developing the individual practitioner by valuing and promoting good practice.

DEFINITIONS OF SUPERVISION

Like the whole concept of 'helping', supervision is not a straightforward process. It is a complex relationship which has very little in terms of a tangible product and it is very difficult to assess its effectiveness (Hawkins and Shohet, 1989). At a kind of macro level, the College of Occupational Therapists (1990) state that it is:

a professional activity which is required at a number of levels, each characterized by a range of tasks. Firstly, it is essential in the planning and delivery of a total programme to an organization or client group. Secondly, it may be centred on the management of a group of staff and the organization of workloads. Thirdly, it is a professional relationship which ensures good standards of practice and encourages professional development (p. 1).

We are particularly concerned, in this context, with the third level described above. Supervision is seen as an interpersonal relationship generally facilitated through the one-to-one interaction of a supervisor and a supervisee, but occasionally enacted through a group process.

PURPOSE OF SUPERVISION

Horton (1993) suggests that it should provide both support and a challenge to the worker's methods of practice, in order to maintain and develop their effectiveness in the given tasks for which they are employed. Nelson (1989) states that the improvements in performance brought about by effective supervision should benefit, in order of importance:

- the organization;
- the individual practitioner;
- the profession.

FUNCTIONS OF SUPERVISION

Hawkins and Shohet (1989) suggest:

> The supervisor has to integrate the role of educator with that of being the provider of support to the worker, and in most cases, managerial oversight of the supervisee's clients. These three functions do not always sit comfortably together ... (p. 4).

We may draw a more detailed list of functions that would fit within the remit of these three broad roles, as follows:

- the maintenance and development of therapeutic competence;
- to monitor effectiveness of helping relationships;
- to oversee the quality and quantity of case load/workload responsibilities;
- to assist with effective management of time;
- to enable professional development, continuing education and training;
- to consider future career development;
- to ensure awareness and effective use of resources;
- to acknowledge effective and successful use of skills;
- to share and explore the emotional demands of other people's psychological difficulties;
- to deal with stress, prevent burnout and address the negative aspects of work;
- to offer support for personal needs and growth.

NEEDS FOR SUPERVISION

Shorrocks and Curran (1994) state that their experience of the occupational therapy profession is one of relative unfamiliarity with the concept of supervision. They pose the question whether supervision is only viewed as a need for new inexperienced staff, that maybe somehow practitioners come to believe that seniority reflects a lesser need for supervision. Their counter-argument to these observations is that an opportunity to stand back and reflect on what we are doing, and how we are doing it, can be of benefit to all practitioners and managers alike. Supervision is an important element of providing a 'quality' service and should be acknowledged as an integral part of the organizational management throughout its entire structure.

Who supervises the supervisor? This is a significant question if we accept the value of this function, contributing to the overall quality of service development, as well as service provision. In a well-defined team hierarchy, responsibility for supervision can reasonably cascade through the structure. However, there is still the question of the overall team manager.

He or she may need to look outside the team or at least accept the value of team clinical and planning meetings as a method of group supervision. This latter suggestion will be influenced by the manager's personal style of leadership.

At the more specific level, in relation to the client group and case management themes of this particular text, a number of important needs for supervision may be identified:

- working with the long-term mentally ill client group is recognized as difficult and demanding work, even seen as unsatisfying work by some practitioners;
- the subgroup of people identified as mentally disorders offenders and/or subject to close 'supervision' present the practitioner with an additional set of tensions and anxieties;
- adopting case management approaches necessitates a fundamental challenge to the traditional organization and practices of multi-disciplinary teams;
- offsetting the potential for staff burnout.

Hawkins and Shohet (1989) remind us of some of the potential consequences of a lack of, resistance to or even inadequate supervision. Practitioners may become professionally quite isolated, with a staleness of approach to their work, rigidity in attitudes and even quite defensive of their practice. Bad and/or habitual practices may become ingrained, standards can drop and reactions to questioning or criticism may border on arrogant denial.

ISSUES ARISING FROM WORKING WITH THE CLIENT GROUP

Staff attitudes and satisfaction

The question of timescale presents a particular concern for many service practitioners. The long-term nature of mental health difficulties generates a need for long-term service involvement, whether continuously or intermittently. This need for a long-term working relationship, spanning years, conflicts with the personal learning and career developments envisaged by many practitioners. Frequently, a service will allow itself to be organized in conjunction with short-term staff placement, enabling them to gain a degree of knowledge and experience in one specialism before moving on to another. However, rapid turnover of staff is often cited as a cause of dissatisfaction for the client.

In conjunction with the issue of timescale is that of the nature of change. Many staff view the client group to be 'chronic' and unchanging, which generates an undermining of expectations and confidence in professional skills, with a resulting dissatisfaction with the work. The changes that occur are often perceived to be very small and extremely slow. It is the function of supervision to help the practitioner adjust their expectations, plan to break down goals to a small scale and to celebrate achievement of individual goals in the spirit of their significance related to a history of relative non-achievement. What seems like a small change to the worker may in fact be quite a major achievement for the service user.

A service-centred focus that defines the individual practitioner's role and expertise more tightly in line with their professional training will generally serve to compound the perception of non-achievement and frustration. A more client-centred approach, encouraging a loosening of professional definitions and an extension of individual roles with the client, enables us to view our work with the individual as much more varied and complex in its scope, offering greater opportunity for reward and satisfaction to the practitioner as well as the service user. This extension of role presents other difficulties for some staff and will be discussed later in the case management approaches.

A further issue in working with the long-term client group is the extent of disturbance and disability that has to be confronted and accepted. Hawkins and Shohet (1989) remind us that: 'The supervisor's role is not just to reassure the worker, but to allow the emotional disturbance to be felt within the safer setting of the supervisory relationship, where it can be survived, reflected upon and learnt from ...' (p. 3).

Empowerment or dependency?

It is easy to fall into the trap of assuming that people with a long history of mental health problems are not capable of organizing and achieving their own goals. Surely, if they could, they would not be in their current position of helplessness? Yet, this standpoint suggests that, if the services had not created a position of dependency, maybe the individual would be empowered to achieve more. We often create dependency through an unintentional undermining of the client's self-worth by our own haste to take control of the situation.

Read and Wallcraft (1992) remind us that it is difficult to empower the client with long-term mental health problems when, as workers or as a service, we often do not feel particularly empowered ourselves. Yet much of the literature on 'strengths' case management (Chapter 3) seeks to challenge this view by enabling the client to become a director of the helping process through the medium of a strong interpersonal relationship with the case manager. Witheridge (1989) suggests that the rights of the service user for self-determination and empowerment are central to good practice and should come before any worker desires to uphold the ideals of 'professional success'. Harris (1990) indicates the significance of the supervisory relationship for helping us to monitor our own professional behaviours on how they affect the balance of creating a dependency or a climate for client autonomy and personal growth.

Working with high-risk clients

The dramatic impacts of incidents of violence, threats of aggression, suicides and self-harming behaviour; the unpleasant atmosphere and conditions of severe neglect; the harrowing details of some offences or behaviours; and the prominence of security and precautions to manage risk; all of these factors have the capacity to dissuade people from engaging in particular areas of work. Indeed, Patmore and Weaver (1992) report evidence to suggest that the unattractive side of this work often leads to practitioners and community teams drifting away from the challenge, unless proper management, direction and supervision can help to focus and support people in the demands encountered. Prins (1986) suggest that the emotional demands and the presenting problems can frequently evoke an 'intangible disquiet and apprehension' in the service practitioner.

Furthermore, the nature of the role may possibly put the practitioner in the unusual position of having to face and support the needs of their own assailant. The demands on the supervisory relationship in this situation would emphasize the need for clear decisions to be made about changing workers or addressing the dual needs of the emotional distress of the original incident and of the return to the circumstances of the incident (Wykes, 1994). Lloyd (1995) stresses the need for training and supervisory support to address:

- education around the management of violence;
- helping the worker assess their own capabilities;
- aspects of 'therapeutic' communication;
- identifying warning signs and sources of stress.

ISSUES ARISING FROM CASE MANAGEMENT APPROACHES

The challenge of a new role

Case management services have been specifically targeted at this client group as a method of developing a different approach from the not-so-successful application of traditional professional boundaries. In an attempt to become more user centred and less service centred, case management demands that individual practitioners make certain fundamental changes.

The traditional values of being a specialist trained within the boundaries of one profession but applying your skills across generic client groups have to be completely turned around. In essence, case management demands that you become a specialist in the client group, but develop a broader, more generalized scope to your skills. For some practitioners, this approach proves too much of a challenge, threatening to isolate them professionally and undermine their application of core skills. For those who feel attracted to invest in the new challenges, the reward is a transferring of expertise from one set of skills to another, with no sense of 'losing' the comfortable feeling of being in possession of a special role.

The central theme of this new role is 'flexibility'. Bleach (1994) describes how participant practitioners in the case management pilot projects valued the flexibility to cross professional boundaries, the flexibility to attend to the wants and needs of individual service users and the flexibility to take the service to where it could be most effective through an outreach perspective. The value of the supervisory relationship lies in its ability to explore the necessary and possible degrees of flexibility whilst at the same time maintaining some kind of 'reality check' on the dangers of misconstruing oneself as the 'all-providing super-therapist'.

Furthermore, in addition to the 'culture of support' that should ideally develop across the team, the supervisory relationship enables practitioners to be more creative in their responses to client needs. This is particularly so in the cases where the client is rejecting offers of services for various reasons (Chapter 5). Creative responses to difficult problems can help motivate the practitioner to persevere. Despite these statements of advantage, many practitioners still have a valid right to defend their own preferences for staying within the boundaries of professional training, where roles can feel safer and more clearly defined.

Case loads

The nature of the work and demanding tasks of focusing on the needs of the long-term and/or high-risk client group have generated much recent debate about case load sizes. If we are targeting the most complex and needy of clients, then by definition the case load size needs to be kept within reasonable limits, e.g. a maximum of 1–15 (Chapter 3). Whilst this suggestion is generally understood, the organization and management across services appears to find it difficult to accommodate effectively.

A specialist case management or intensive outreach team has the advantages of being able to more clearly define its boundaries and target client group; it may be able to develop its supportive culture across the team because of a common focus and shared interest in the specific tasks of the team and it may be able to become more responsive and creative for its client group, because of the elimination of competing demands on its resources. However, it falls out of favour with many managers because of its clear short-term high financial costs and it evokes a separation and defensiveness from other associated services because of the perception that it is challenging the existing well-developed practices of other teams.

Generic community mental health teams present a different set of complex issues when looking at the case load implications. If we seek to spread clients of this particular group into small numbers across everybody's case load, we set up conditions for varying qualities of service response, at best, as the degree of interest and expertise in the needs of this client will vary between different workers. At worst, we set the more usual conditions for all of these clients to receive a reduced level of service as competing demands and the inevitable attraction towards the sources of quicker results take time away from the people who present with complex and needy circumstances.

The task for the supervisory relationship becomes one of helping individual practitioners to carefully manage their case loads, through linking weightings of need to levels of contact. However, we need to acknowledge that the end product is far less simple than this statement may imply, as numerous extraneous factors such as wider support network, crisis management and client choice will all influence decisions for the ongoing management of a case load.

Discharge or disengagement

The very nature of the needs of the client group and the complexity of individual personal history suggest that discharging people is not usually a satisfactory outcome. Yet case load sizes cannot increase indefinitely. It is reasonable, however, to expect that many people achieve sufficient benefit from long-term contact with a service to allow the frequency of contact to be gradually diminished to reflect greater independence and user empowerment (Kisthardt, 1992). Many people cope extremely well in the knowledge that a service can be easily and quickly accessed, without necessarily having to maintain a high level of direct contact. It is often the formality and perceived finality of the term 'discharge' that can invoke a sense of failing and dependency.

The supervisory relationship can be proactive in monitoring the gradual reduction of contact levels and if the process of discharge is effected, the practitioner can be encouraged to offer the client information on how a service can be reaccessed in future need, though this latter point should reasonably be more prominent in team policy rather than individual supervision.

Line and professional management

The multiprofessional role and multidisciplinary constituency of case management teams challenges the traditional concept of management responsibility through the hierarchy of a single profession. The main source of tension arises between the need to maintain high 'profession-based' standards and the need to be more flexible and responsive to diverse client needs. This tension will manifest itself at a service level through local power struggles between the management of different professions. It will also manifest itself for the individual practitioner through the need to develop a multiprofessional perspective on client needs and the perceived threat to the performance of core skills.

The difficult resolution of these tensions lies in the team manager, from any profession, taking responsibility for issues of day-to-day management and supervision, including the promotion of the multiprofessional roles. Team members from a different profession than that of their line manager should have access to clearly defined lines of professional management and support from outside the team. Ideally, the access of outside support should be at the discretion of the individual team member, rather than enforced by the professional manager from outside. An efficiently functioning system will be more responsive to client and staff needs if it is less controlled by the competing agendas of different external hierarchies.

ISSUES OF STAFF BURNOUT

Definition

A state of physical, emotional and mental exhaustion, resulting from an extended period of intense involvement with people who are very emotionally demanding (Pines, 1982). Hawkins and Shohet (1989) suggest it:

... is not an illness that you catch, neither is it a recognizable event or state, for it is a process that often begins very early in one's career as a helper. Indeed its seeds may be inherent in the belief systems of many of the helping professions and in the personalities of those that are attracted to them (p. 20).

It is generally characterized by physical fatigue, feelings of helplessness and hopelessness, negative self-worth, negative attitudes towards other staff and clients', feelings of guilt, failure, inadequacy and incompetence. It may also be identified through a mid-career sense of apathy and disinterest in learning and developing professionally, where a practitioner resorts to relying on set patterns of activity and behaviour, almost unthinkingly.

Causes and prevention

Extensive lists of factors may be identified as contributors to burnout, with a focus on the perceived pressures of the job and lack of managerial support and direction (Onyett et al., 1995). Lloyd (1995) identifies these under the negative aspects of the following subheadings:

- work overload;
- work underload;
- work variety;
- work isolation;
- work significance;
- work activity;
- work position;
- work efficiency;
- work role conflict;
- work social support;
- work supervisors;
- work feedback;
- work environments.

Burnout may clearly be seen as a consequence of poor supervision. Conversely, a well-developed supervisory relationship provides an essential foundation for preventing burnout. Hawkins and Shohet (1989) suggest it should be attended to before it happens, through examining our own motivations for working in the helping professions, monitoring our own symptoms of stress, creating an environment for learning throughout our careers and developing a balanced life outside our 'helping' activities. Onyett et al. (1995) report an extensive study that draws our attention to the perceived rewards that promote job satisfaction in a wide range of community mental health teams.

The supervisory relationship may also provide a primary focus for examining our work expectations, our development of relationships with service users, the flexibility and creativity of our approaches and the potential impact of burnout through work practices (Bleach, 1994).

THE SKILLS OF SUPERVISION

Application of counselling skills

Hawkins and Shohet (1989) identify many of the qualities that make an effective supervisor as being the essential skills of counselling: '... empathy, understanding, unconditional positive regard, congruence, genuineness, warmth, self-disclosure, flexibility, concern, attention, investment, curiosity and openness' (p. 35). Indeed, the general conditions and environment are the same as would be expected of a formal counselling session, in terms of the space, furnishing, atmosphere and focus on verbal and non-verbal behaviours.

Horton (1993) suggests that supervision may sometimes blur into the realms of personal counselling, but whilst this need not be discouraged it is important to clearly acknowledge the boundary between the two functions. Supervision should frequently employ the skills of counselling, but whereas counselling is essentially an approach directed at the emotional content of the client engaged within the present relationship, supervision will have a practical structure for exploring the work within relationships that exist outside the supervision session.

'Feedback' is a significant counselling skill employed within the supervisory relationship. Stengelhofen (1993) suggests that it is the essential information that a supervisor provides to help the supervisee adjust their working practices in order to achieve or re-evaluate their stated goals. To be of utmost value it needs to be immediate in its delivery but also to sustain the active involvement of the supervisee it should evolve continuous and collaborative qualities.

A further element of counselling practice that promotes good quality supervision is the establishment of a supervisory contract. Horton (1993) suggests that a contract is essential to establish the more formal boundaries of supervision, to prevent it drifting into the more casual conversations about work that frequently take place between work colleagues on an entirely informal basis. An essential element of such a contract is its mutual negotiation, as different people have very different experiences and expectations of what supervision is all about. The contract may be a written or a verbal agreement, but should address:

- place and frequency of contact (2–4 weekly being average);
- the required or permitted functions: professional practice, career development, personal issues;

- confidentiality of spoken and any written information;
- process of appraisal and review of the supervisory relationship;
- procedures for resolving issues of 'difference' in the relationship.

Encouraging self-awareness

Similar to the concept of feedback, the development of self-awareness should be a gradual and continuous process, which may be facilitated in part by the interactions in the supervisory relationship. Burnard (1992) suggests that a fuller awareness of self enables us to have a sharper and clearer understanding of what is happening to others. This quality is obviously just as applicable to the supervisor as it is to the super-visee.

Self-awareness should ideally begin with an exploration of our own motives for becoming professional 'helpers'. Hawkins and Shohet (1989) highlight the dangers that may lie in the very personality of people attracted to the helping professions, particularly adhering to the illusion that we have some special qualities which we impart to 'needy others'.

Bleach (1994) reminds us that it is often difficult or even painful to acknowledge causes for dysfunction that may arise out of our own personality or working practices but a good supervisory relationship may help to address these issues.

Exploring staff attitudes

We have already acknowledged that for some individuals the concept of supervision is viewed with some scepticism. The supervisor needs to be aware of the potential sources of blocking to effective supervision:

- supervisee's previous experiences of supervision;
- personal inhibitions about disclosing details of working practice;
- inherent factors in the supervisory relationship, e.g. personal, sexual, cultural;
- resistance to the implied formality;
- pressures of work wrongly relegating the priority for supervision;
- perceiving the negative implications of scrutiny;
- general apathy and ambivalence associated with burnout.

Stengelhofen (1993) suggests that the innate attitudes towards 'professionalism', including professional practice and relationships, have a much stronger influence than the individual's theoretical and practical knowledge base. The idea of supervision is somehow linked with the broader issues of professionalism and the effectiveness of the supervisory relationship may be consequently influenced by such attitudes. The implication for the supervisor is one of maintaining staff development through continuing opportunities for education and training high on the supervisee's agenda. These opportunities should not simply focus on developments in clinical practice but also on career development, managerial, organizational, ethical and professional issues.

A further aspect of professional development is highlighted by Nelson (1989) when he suggests that the encouragement of individuality has potentially positive and negative energies. The negative side becomes evident where the individual practitioner loses sight of the main aims of the organization or team. The difficulty for the manager or supervisor lies in judging where non-conformity can be constructive and creative, opening new visions of achieving the objectives. Nelson reminds us that enforcing uniformity only leads to stultifying imagination, initiative and energy.

FORMALITY AND INFORMALITY

The above discussion implies that supervision takes place within a formalized contractual agreement, where two people meet face to face at agreed intervals to discuss specific aspects of the supervisee's clinical and professional development. This is the most clearly understood method of implementing supervision.

However, for working with this particularly demanding and needy client group, the time interval between supervision sessions may not be responsive to the individual practitioner's need for spontaneous unloading of emotional content. Whilst impromptu supervision sessions may occasionally be arranged at short notice, the overall workload demands generally render this response impossible. For this reason, amongst others, it becomes vitally important that the team is organized in such a way that a 'culture of support' may be engendered.

A more informal but equally effective culture of support is reflected by each team member being available as a 'sounding board' or being in tune with the emotional demands of their colleagues' case loads. Within reasonable boundaries of professionalism and confidentiality, a team member should feel able to celebrate their client achievements or share the occasional trauma and despondency with colleagues in the office. Similarly, team members should attend to the pressures and demands of colleagues and feel able to enquire tactfully into the potential build-up of pressures.

The informality of support should be additional to the formal supervisory relationship and should reflect in spontaneous offers of back-up or co-working where needed. Finally, we should not overlook the value of humour as a vitally important element of support. Particularly in the face of traumatic and emotionally demanding work, the appropriate use of humour within a staff team should act as an effective pressure release, individually and collectively. It should not be devalued as unprofessional, as a perpetually serious approach can only result in burnout.

GROUP SUPERVISION

This discussion has focused entirely on the individual supervisory relationship, in line with the overall theme of this text. However, we should acknowledge that a great deal of formal supervision also takes place in groups, through clinical review meetings or facilitated staff support groups.

The strengths model of case management has also developed its own unique approach to group supervision (Rapp and Kisthardt, 1991). This is a method of improving the effectiveness of the clinical review meeting through achieving:

- affirmation: the recognition of the work being undertaken;
- information: the sharing and clarifying of details;
- ideas: generating new options;
- fun: to ensure colleagues in a team are enjoying the work.

Essentially this approach is a peer-based sharing of a strengths-orientated process. It involves active listening, validating different opinions and viewpoints and a brainstorming of ideas around any defined clinical situation. An essential requirement is to keep the process personal, in the here and now, not distracted by abstract professional concepts. The brainstorming element should encourage creativity; even the wildest of spontaneous ideas can be validated for their contribution to 'fun' and their potential to trigger the thoughts of others. Personal curiosity and inventiveness have a role in keeping the process fresh and positive.

SUMMARY

Clients presenting with long-term problems and high degrees of risk are a very needy group of people, who present the practitioner with a complex range of issues and tasks and intense emotional demands. In this light, Hawkins and Shohet (1989) suggest that staff supervision becomes a valuable part of taking care of oneself, maintaining a commitment to learning and addressing the issues of self-awareness and ongoing professional and personal development. Within the supervisory relationship, the supervisor is required to integrate supportive, educational and managerial roles.

Nelson (1989) reminds us that some staff greet supervision with ambivalence, concerned about degrees of scrutiny and criticism.

However, good supervision should be seen as promoting good practice and as an invaluable method for counteracting the destructiveness of staff burnout in the face of repetitive, difficult and emotionally demanding work.

The skills of supervision are essentially an adaptation of counselling skills and it is a function that may be performed in individual or group settings. Shorrocks and Curran (1994) state that if we believe supervision to be essential to the provision of a high quality service, then it should be an acknowledged and respected activity central to the organizational framework of a team or service.

REFERENCES

Bleach, A. (1994) *'Engagement' Draft Training Module'*, Research and Development for Psychiatry, London.

Burnard, P. (1992) *Communication Skills for Health Professionals*, Chapman & Hall, London.

College of Occupational Therapists (1990) *Standards, Policies and Proceedings: Statement on Supervision in Occupational Therapy,* College of Occupational Therapists, London.

Harris, M. (1990) Redesigning case management services for work with character disordered young adult patients, in *Psychiatry Takes to the Streets*, (ed. N.L. Cohen), Guilford Press, New York, pp. 156–76.

Hawkins, P. and Shohet, R. (1989) *Supervision in the Helping Professions*, Open University Press, Buckingham.

Horton, I. (1993) Supervision, in *Counselling and Psychology for Health Professionals*, (eds R. Bayne and P. Nicolson), Chapman & Hall, London, pp. 15–33.

Kisthardt, W.E. (1992) A strengths model of case management: the principles and functions of a helping partnership with persons with persistent mental illness, in *A Strengths Perspective for Social Work Practice,* (ed. D. Saleeby), Longman, New York, pp. 59–83.

Lloyd, C. (1995) *Forensic Psychiatry for Health Professionals,* Chapman & Hall, London.

Nelson, M.J. (1989) *Managing Health Professionals*, Chapman & Hall, London.

Onyett, S., Pillinger, T. and Muijen, M. (1995) *Making Community Mental Health Teams Work,* Sainsbury Centre for Mental Health, London.

Patmore, C. and Weaver, T. (1992) Improving community services for serious mental disorder. *Journal of Mental Health,* 1, 107–15.

Pines, A. (1982) Helpers motivation and the burnout syndrome, in *Basic Processes in Helping Relationships,* (ed. T.A. Wills), Academic Press, New York.

Prins, H. (1986) *Dangerous Behaviour: The Law and Mental Disorder*, Tavistock, London.

Rapp, C.A. and Kisthardt, W.E. (1991) RDP Pilot Case Management Projects. Workshop on the Strengths Model. Hoddesdon, November.

Read, J. and Wallcraft, J. (1992) *Guidelines for Empowering Users of Mental Health Services*, MIND and COHSE, London.

Shorrocks, J. and Curran, A. (1994) Supervision for occupational therapy staff. *Occupational Therapy News*, **2**(1), 7.

Stengelhofen, J. (1993) *Teaching Students in Clinical Settings*, Chapman & Hall, London.

Witheridge, T.F. (1989) The assertive community treatment worker: an emerging role and its implications for professional training. *Hospital and Community Psychiatry*, **40**(6), 620–4.

Wykes, T. (ed.) (1994) *Violence and Health Care Professionals*, Chapman & Hall, London.

FURTHER READING

Cherniss, C. (1981) *Staff Burnout: Job Stress in the Human Services*, Sage, London.

Houston, G. (1990) *Supervision and Counselling*, Rochester Foundation, London.

Index